30 Days of Inducing

The Complete Guide to Making Breast Milk in One Month

Jennifer Elisabeth Maiden

INTRODUCTION

How to Make Breast Milk in One Month:
A Step by Step Guide

Mr. S and I have been a nursing couple for almost as long as we've been married, and throughout the course of our relationship, which has spanned nearly 18 years, we have experienced nursing in all of its beautiful forms--from maternal to dry; when we decided to re-dedicate our ANR (which, in our case, meant agreeing that we would once more commit to being a "nightly nursing couple" rather than the occasional sucklers that life's sweet transitions had sort of forced us to become), the idea of nursing with breast milk didn't come into the initial discussion. While opening these lines of communication, he and I found that we had both missed the intimate connection of our once-frequent nursing sessions, but what we didn't realize was that he and I also shared a private desire: we wanted to pursue lactation. By then, we had been dry nursing about one to four times per month following the weaning of our youngest child for a little over five years, and I absolutely loved every minute of it, but every time Mr. S would fall asleep following a suckling session, I would lie awake, wondering if it could actually be possible for me to produce non-maternal breast milk. It was an intriguing idea, one that remained private, but every so often, I would find myself drawn to the internet, always in search of an answer that I never found.

At that point, I was only beginning to realize that what Mr. S and I had shared for so long had a name (ANR), and that there were others like us "out there", so I found myself spending time on traditional breastfeeding sites and forums, poring through pages of data. Unless you're lucky enough to stumble across a post from an adult nurser (or an adoptive mother), these forums aren't the best places to find information on inducing and re-lactation, and when I was able to find this information, most of it was scattered, archived, and really dated. I read it anyway, and it was not promising.

Did you ever notice that the question *Can a woman make breast milk if she isn't pregnant?* typically returns two definitive answers?

1. No.
2. Yes, but she has to take medication to make it happen.

0/10 on the Helpful Scale.

I didn't like those answers at all, and can you imagine where I would be now, nearly 2 1/2 years later, if I had taken them at face value rather than with a grain of salt?

The search continued.

I finally found a snippet of information on inducing lactation that set me on the right track-- and would be much more compatible with my lifestyle than the other advice I'd read about around-the-clock pumping and manual stimulation, combined with difficult-to-obtain medications, which I absolutely did not have time for--or any interest in. The basic idea behind being able to produce breast milk in one month involved a minimum of one carefully timed nursing session per day, so I decided to use that sketchy concept as a basis for my own journey into re-lactation, and believe it or not, it actually worked. As time went on, I began to talk to my friend Holly, a Labor and Delivery RN, who introduced me to a small group of lactation consultants, the lovely ladies I still work closely with, and have now been able to share and exchange information with another close friend, an adoptive mother who has been able to produce a sufficient amount of milk for not just one, but two bundles of joy. (Interesting note: she uses the same techniques as many adult nursing women, including a carefully timed daily inducing routine that includes massage, pumping, TENS Unit stimulation, and a cocktail of fenugreek and blessed thistle.)

People will say that there's a huge difference between maternal lactation and induced lactation. The confusing truth to this is that there is...but there isn't. Lactation is lactation-- and it's just as much emotional as it is physical. The intimate closeness of your ANR will take care of the emotional aspects by setting key hormones (such as oxytocin and prolactin) necessary to the milk-making process into place; this step-by-step guide will assist you with the physical facets. By combining the two, lactation is a very real possibility for every woman, regardless of her age or stage in life.

I've often been asked how I achieved lactation so quickly. While I did become fully lactated in a little over 3 1/2 months, the supply building and maintaining process that followed has been a true labor of love, one that has taken about 15 months to achieve. (One of the best investments I've ever made!)
While it's good to know that breast milk can be made in just 30 days, it's wonderful to know how it's done, so I present to you this honest, practical, and relatively simple step-by-step guide that I (and now several other women) have successfully followed as a way to get that liquid gold flowing! You don't need a lot of fancy things or an inducing arsenal to make this work. Essentially, 30 Days of Inducing only requires three basic things:

1.   A willing (and properly suckling) mouth
2.   Approximately 90 minutes of time
3.   Determination and commitment

A good-quality breast pump helps, but it isn't necessary. I induced with fantastic results for the first five weeks of my re-lactation journey, relying on nothing more than Mr. S and my own two hands to get the job done! But in case you are interested in investing in a pump, I've included the "Best Breast Pump List" series and my review of the Spectra S2 breast pump at the end of this book.

Many factors contribute to a woman's individual lactation success. When I began my personal re-lactation journey:

- I had exclusively and extensively breastfed three children, all who self-weaned at approximately 30 months of age.
- I had been dry for a little over five years.
- Aside from keeping a close watch on my potential for anemia, I had no other pre-existing medical conditions.
- My prolactin levels tend to run slightly higher than normal. (I have always produced a lot (and by a lot, I mean enormous amounts) of breast milk.)
- I had not undergone hysterectomy.
- I was not taking any prescription medications.
- My body was not undergoing any of the three stages of menopause.
- I was not using any form of birth control.

While none of these factors make or break inducing/re-lactation success, it's still important to take them into consideration, as some conditions change the inducing process; they don't necessarily prevent the process from happening, but they can slow it down, or be contributing factors to the amount of milk that's being produced.

The basics of 30 Days are quite simple.

1. You need to commit to this program by following the included 30-day guide as close to exactly as you possibly can.
2. The key to success is scheduling.

Choose inducing time(s) that you can strictly adhere to for 1 full month. Do not vary from your chosen, or "set", time(s). This carefully regulated schedule helps your body to recognize a need for breast milk.

Sometimes, adult nursing couples need to arrange their inducing routine around pressing daily activities and responsibilities. It's fine to take a practical approach to this; after all, we're busy people, right? Just induce when the time is right for you. In my case, my "best" inducing times were 6 a.m., 2 p.m., and 11 p.m. This is the schedule I have adhered to since March 27, 2016.

If something comes up and you can't induce at your set time, always remember that life happens and that is okay. Don't stress, over-think, or feel guilty. Induce as soon as possible, and get right back on track the next day! It's helpful if you can induce no more than 1.5-2 hours prior to or following your set time.

An example of this would be a set time of 9 a.m. in which you aren't able to induce at that exact moment. You can arrange your schedule to induce as early as 7:30 a.m. or as late as 11:00 a.m. without harming routine. (Just do this as infrequently as possible, and try to limit this to a maximum of three times during the 30-day inducing process.)

Knowing how to nurse correctly is vital. Nursing involves suckling; this is gentle, but rhythmic oral massage of the areolae, and much different from traditional forms of sexualized breast play and stimulation. You cannot stimulate milk production and flow by sucking on a nipple. (Let's be honest, this feels *ah-may-ZING*, but it isn't conducive to successful lactation.) Before you can suckle, you will also need to know how to properly latch. Both work in perfect harmony to produce, build, and maintain breast milk supply. Even in the adult nursing relationship, latching and suckling difficulties are typically what impedes inducing most often, and many couples find that once this issue is corrected, the process goes along a lot more smoothly.

Basic Inducing Tips:

1. If possible, perform 1 inducing method in the morning. Just like the rest of our bodies, our breasts have a way of responding to milk-making much more effectively in the morning after a good night's sleep!
2. Space your inducing sessions out as much as you can through the day. Always allow at least 1 hour in between inducing sessions to allow your breasts to rejuvenate and replenish.
3. Warmth and moisture often help to stimulate the breasts and prep them for inducing and expression. Before inducing, apply moist warm compresses to the breasts, or massage in the shower or while bathing. You can even use a heating pad set on low against your back or shoulders while nursing or pumping. (This actually feels really nice and relaxing!)
4. Always stay as calm and relaxed as possible. Focus on your lactation goals, but don't stress about them. STRESS IMPEDES LACTATION. (And we don't want that!)
5. Drink 4 ounces of water prior to inducing, and drink another 4 ounces immediately after.

How to Use 30 Days of Inducing for the Adult Nursing Couple

The program will include:

- A minimum of 1 nursing session per day.
- A minimum of 1 manual/massage session per day.
- A minimum of 1 pumping session per day.

1. Specific techniques will be listed in detail under each daily inducing checklist.
2. If you do not have a breast pump, replace a typical pumping session with either nursing or massage.

Women often ask if they can perform more inducing sessions than the 30 Days protocol recommends, and the question is quite simple to answer. Of course, although it isn't necessary. 30 Days will work as it is written, but some women prefer to induce more frequently through the day. Adding sessions is perfectly fine (as long as you schedule them), but subtracting? Well...not so much. Even if you choose to take a more minimalist approach to inducing, follow the basic 30 Days plan as it is described in this guide to maximize success.

How to Use 30 Days of Inducing for the Occasional Nurser

The program will include:

- A minimum of 4 nursing sessions in the 30-day period of time.
- A minimum of 2-3 non-nursing sessions per day. (This will depend on whether or not you're suckling)

If you only nurse occasionally, you'll need to rely on other forms of inducing to get your milk flowing, and this will consist of pumping and/or manual stimulation at least 3 times a day. Set a goal to nurse at least once per week during the month.

On nursing days, you will include:

- A minimum of 1 daily suckling session.
- A minimum of 1 daily manual/massage session.
- A minimum of 1 pumping session per day. (You might find it particularly helpful to power pump.

Details on this inducing method will be included in individual daily checklists.

On non-nursing (or off) days, you will perform a minimum of 3 alternative inducing techniques on the day(s) you do not nurse. If doing this, your best option will be to perform 2 manual/massage sessions and 1 power pumping session per day.

How to Use 30 Days of Inducing for the Self-Inducing Woman

The program will include:

- A minimum of three carefully timed inducing sessions per day.

Self-inducing suggestions:

1. Perform 1 power pumping session, 1 manual/massage session, and end with 1 power pumping session per day.
2. Perform 1 manual/massage session followed by 2 power pumping sessions per day.
3. Perform 2 manual/massage sessions followed by 1 power pumping session per day.
4. Each should be spaced at least 1 hour apart.

Quick Nursing Tip:

A great nursing session involves a minimum of 40 minutes of effective suckling. This includes 20 minutes of suckling on each breast.

Quick Manual/Massage Tip:

Depending on the form of manual stimulation you choose, and whether or not you induce your breasts individually or simultaneously, effective massage will take between 15 and 40 minutes to perform.

Quick Pumping Tips:

1. If using a traditional form of pumping with a single pump kit, this method of inducing will take 40 minutes to perform. (This includes 20 minutes of stimulation per breast)
2. If using a traditional form of pumping with a double pump kit, this method of inducing will take 20 minutes to perform.
3. If power pumping, using either a single or double pumping kit, this inducing method will take 1 hour to perform.
4. If you will be providing stimulation with a manual pump, information on how to do so efficiently and effectively is included in this guide.

Optional Inducing Methods:

1. Nipple Stimulation

It can be very beneficial to perform nipple stimulation prior to at least 1 of your daily inducing methods.

To Properly Stimulate Your Nipples:

1. Stimulate one erect nipple at a time.
2. Using your thumb and index finger, begin by grasping your right nipple at the base where it connects to the areola, and pull gently downward.
3. Roll your nipple between your thumb and finger for 1 minute.
4. Rest for 2-4 minutes.
5. Move to the left nipple. Repeat steps 2-4.
6. Stimulate each nipple for a total of 5 minutes.

2. TENS Unit Stimulation

A TENS Unit can be worn throughout the day, and used for 15 minutes every two hours, in between traditional inducing methods, to provide additional breast stimulation.

How to Use a Double Channel TENS Unit for Breast Stimulation:

Stand in front of a mirror and use one channel for your left breast and the second channel for your right breast. The pads will be marked to identify a positive (+) electrode and a negative (-) electrode.

Beginning with your left breast, apply the positive electrode to your breast, approximately one inch from the side of your nipple, and then apply the negative pad directly across from it, one inch from the opposite side of your nipple. Repeat this process with the second channel, placing the pads on either side of your right nipple. When looking in the mirror, the unit's channels, electrodes, and your nipples should be well-aligned, and it should look something like this:

+Electrode (breast) Left nipple (breast) -Electrode (cleavage) -Electrode (breast) Right nipple (breast) +Electrode, or:

(+ o -) (- o +), which signifies the proper electrode placement and alignment when looking in a mirror.

Once the pads are in place, you can get dressed and begin stimulation simply by turning on the unit and adjusting its wave, amplitude, pulse, frequency, and/or intensity to suit your individual needs.

3. Breast Compressions

To perform breast compressions:

Once you and your partner have settled into a comfortable nursing position and he is properly latched to the breast, allow him to suckle for approximately five minutes to encourage the let-down reflex. You can then incorporate your first set of breast compressions.

To provide proper compressions, curve your hand into a C-shape, allowing the side of your breast to rest comfortably in the cupped palm of your hand with your fingers supporting the underside of the breast and resting against the wall of the chest. Your thumb will lie flat along the top of the areola, and help to provide pressure during this technique. Your thumb should not press into the areola, as this can inhibit milk flow; when performing compressions, be sure not to disturb your partner's latch. If he does come off the breast, help him re-latch, and then re-position your hand.

Firmly squeeze your breast. Your fingers will push upward while your thumb presses down, and the breast will flatten slightly. Hold the position for five minutes as your partner suckles, then release. The release allows your hand and breast to rest. Your partner should continue to nurse during this rest

After five minutes have gone by, apply a second five-minute set of breast compressions if you wish, and repeat the process (compress-rest) for the length of the entire nursing session. You can compress either one or both breasts. Compressions is a technique that doesn't require a great deal of consistency, so you don't need to use them during every nursing session, as skipping compressions will not adversely affect breast milk production in any way.

This same technique can be used during pumping, too. Once your breast pump is in place, simply follow the steps listed above to aid in the lactation process. This technique is referred to as Pump Compressions.

While many women enjoy using herbal supplements along with their traditional daily inducing routines, they aren't necessary (and neither are prescription medications used to produce breast milk). Aside from testing out a topical fenugreek poultice (which you can find in my book *DIY Boobie Boosters*) during a recent round of power pumping, I've never incorporated herbal lactogenics into my daily inducing routine. I do recommend taking a daily pre-natal vitamin. While there isn't evidence that these will help you produce more milk, they do seem to aid in the process by providing a good balance of vitamins and minerals that enrich our bodies--and our milk supply.

If you're planning to use herbal supplements to aid in the inducing process, choose the ones you feel will work best for you, and use them in proper combination and/or dosage for the entire 30 days. (Unless you feel that you're having an adverse reaction to them, don't alter the combination in any way.) A Fountain of Gardens, which you can find on the Bountiful Fruits website, is a good herbal supplement reference book.

Other Tips and Information You Might Find Helpful:

1. Adjusting This Plan to Work For You

When I first started devising 30 Days of Inducing, I created it to work around my daily schedule, which always seems to be crazy hectic! I had to time my inducing sessions around my activities, and I could only do a maximum of three sessions without making a lot of compromise. It became pretty simple; I scheduled appointments and errands so they didn't conflict with inducing responsibilities, and if something came up, I made minor adjustments to my schedule. Because some women work outside of the home and because we all have different daily routines and priorities, creating 30 Days for everyone had to provide a lot of flexibility.

The basic plan, which you will find to include a combination of 3 daily inducing methods, can be used as it's written, or you can repeat the pattern throughout the day.   Some women have the time to induce around the clock, and if it works for you and this is something you feel comfortable with doing, then go for it! The core of 30 Days relies mostly on training your body to make milk by regulating your daily schedule. It's important to follow the suggestions of how to correctly take your supplements, the methods you'll use on each specific day, and the length of time you'll induce, but how often you choose to induce is entirely up to you.

When I first began the re-lactation process, I had just about one paragraph of information to go on. And I just went with it. Mr. S and I started our journey with just one effective nursing session, and I was making colostrum in 48 hours. I couldn't believe it! It just seemed too good to be true! That's when I decided to add 1 massage session in the afternoon. Things progressed, and since that was going so well, and we were having such a good time, we added a second nursing session to my inducing routine.
I wanted to keep 30 Days of Inducing *that* simple so all women could comfortably induce without feeling pressure or the time crunch.

And here's an interesting fact that you don't often read about inducing: You absolutely can over-stimulate your breasts.

You know that feeling you get when you're overworked? That *Ugh, I'm so over this thing*? Your breasts can reach that point, too, and if they do, they will automatically close down the milk making process until they feel the time has come to begin working once more. (It's like a Boobie Strike!) There's such a fine line between stimulation and over stimulation.
If something doesn't seem to be working for you, it might be time to change things up a bit, and that can be scary because nobody wants to lose the progress they've made.

It's hard for me to make definitive suggestions on what you "should" do because your body is unique, and will respond to lactation in its own special way; how you use 30 Days is one of those personal judgment calls, but here are some thoughts on making the plan a true success:

- If you've been inducing (or are currently inducing) more than three times a day, and you really don't feel that you're progressing, go ahead and give the 30 Days plan a try. Give your breasts some well-deserved R & R, and monitor your response and reaction to the decreased sessions. If you think you need to increase, then do so.
- If you're using a TENS throughout the day, in between your inducing techniques, then your breasts are getting a lot of additional hands-free deep tissue and areolar stimulation, which can provide peace of mind.
- Your body is probably responding better than you think it is. Remember: your breasts will ONLY make as much milk as they feel you "need".

I *can* promise you that every technique provided in the 30 Days plan has proven effective, and all are the best choices in inducing methods.
By following the basic outline, you simply make the program work for you.

As you read over 30 Days, you'll notice that every day of inducing offers a new manual massage technique, and the reason behind this is really simple: by mixing things up a bit, we can keep our breasts "interested" and responsive while being sure that we're stimulating every inch of the tissue, glands, ducts, and nerves that are vital to the lactation process! Each technique is proven to be a most effective form of natural stimulation--and they're the ones that I've personally used throughout the course of my re-lactation journey.

On days that you'll be performing multiple massage sessions, use that day's technique each time you stimulate; for example, if it's Marnet Day, do only Marmet.

Mixing things up also prevents monotony, and keeping things interesting can help us stay on the right track!

You know the saying, *It's the same stuff, just a different day*? That's pretty much what effective inducing is all about: repetitive measures.

To make milk your breasts need to believe that there is a need for milk--no matter who your recipient is. (And it's nice to know that our breasts are judgment free zones, isn't it? They don't mind if you're nursing an adult; they'll produce milk for anyone. It's just a part of their "job description"!) Not only are we training our breasts to make milk during the first 30 days of inducing, we're conditioning them on how to do so. And, yes, we do this through repetition.

.I think this is one reason that couples stop nursing, or women give up on inducing. I've been told the process is boring. And I suppose it could be to some; it just depends on how you look at it, and how important lactation is to you. Some people dive head first into the waters of ANR with unrealistic expectations, not really realizing how hard this can be. It's definitely a commitment. And it's so awful when nursers get discouraged by the monotony of daily inducing and just give up on the idea of sharing an ANR because they believe that, without breast milk, there can't be nursing, and that could not be further from the truth. Dry nursing is amazing. I highly recommend it!

The first few days of inducing are fun; it's all so new, and everything new is exciting. By the second week, some of that newness wears off, and you might even find yourself thinking, Oh, no. Not again. That's okay...don't feel bad if you start to feel inducing burnout. It happens, but don't quit. You can do this. Mr. S' big philosophy is *After 21 days, anything can become a habit*, and I think that honestly holds true with nursing and inducing, too. You sort of just get "used" to it, and the process becomes another (fabulous) part of your daily routine. By the third week, it's no longer Oh, no. Not again. It becomes, Ooops, gotta run. It's inducing time! And it feels wonderful when you reach that phase!

Basically, if you hope to make milk, repetition is just one of those realities you'll have to face, and it's a lot easier to handle the "induce-and-repeat" pattern if you're truly into the experience. A lot of our success depends on how much we want it.

Oh, and how you view the experience can make a huge difference, too! Don't think of inducing as a routine, think of it as a rhythm--and then get into it! And, instead of thinking, Here I go again, wake up motivated, and ask yourself, Hmm, I wonder what's going to happen today? Staying positive can honestly change our perspective on anything!

Prescription Medications (for Pre-existing Medical Conditions)

Even if you feel that a medication (including birth control) may be negatively affecting your lactation endeavor, do not stop taking it without consulting a qualified medical professional beforehand. It's also important to note that some herbs can negatively interact with certain prescription medications (including estrogens and birth control). Continue any HRT as prescribed by your doctor.

Your Cycle May Affect Nursing and Nursing May Affect Your Cycle

During your period, you may believe that you aren't progressing, or even notice an initial decrease in your milk supply. This is normal--don't stop inducing!
Nursing can cause a change in your cycle; it may become irregular until your body adapts to its new state of lactation (even in the earliest stage), and your flow may either increase or decrease. Unless you're trying to conceive, be cautious with your birth control!

Massage Tips:

1 Oils

Massaging with lactogenic oils is totally optional, but can feel very nice, and not only do they soothe and nourish the delicate skin of the breasts, they can be beneficial to the inducing process. When massaging, most women reach immediately for the coconut oil, but you can try a variety of oils in your daily inducing routine, including apricot, avocado, olive, and grape seed. Coconut oil can cause rash or eczema flares in people with sensitive skin, so discontinue its use if you notice any adverse side effects. A great (and effective) two-ingredient massage oil can be blended at home by adding 1/2 teaspoon of pure aloe vera (not the 99% variety available in retail stores) gel to 1 teaspoon of carrier oil. Warm the blend in the palms of your hands and use it during daily breast massage techniques.

2. Rotations

When performing any sort of circular motion massage on the breast and/or areola, as you will do when using many of the manual techniques listed in this guide, always start at the top. Imagine a clock is printed on your areola; the starting point would be 12:00. Begin your massage at 12 and work around the clock until you reach 12 once more. This is 1 rotation.

3. Additional "Boobie Boosters"

A boobie booster is simply a breast enhancing poultice, mask, cream, or toner that can be used 2-3 times per week in conjunction with your traditional inducing methods as a means of further improving the overall health and beauty of your breasts while working to encourage breast milk production and flow. Many of these recipes can be found in The *Loving Milk Maid's DIY Boobie Boosters*, but I've included some of my personal favorites for you in this guide.

Clean Green Lactation™:

Diet and nutrition are absolutely key to successful lactation! I truly believe that nature's finest super foods (particularly those from the green foods color chart) play an enormous-- and invaluable--part in the inducing/maintaining process. I was practicing a clean eating lifestyle (and still am, as a matter of fact) when I began inducing, and over time, have been working with lactation consultants, my personal physician, and a certified herbalist to create and promote Clean Green Lactation. Do your best to include one healthy, well-balanced meal selection to your daily inducing routine. I'll share various breast-boosting recipes throughout the course of 30 Days of Inducing. Some are taken from my cookbook, others from my personal collection.

Super Foods and Snack Tips:

Green is a beautiful color. It represents life, renewal, nature, and energy, and is associated with all things spring and summer: growth, harmony, freshness, safety, and fertility. It is also the color of some of the best nutrient-enriched fruits and vegetables you could possibly eat, so, when in doubt, go green!

Not only do they provide lactogenic benefits, the low-calorie and high-fiber content of these foods allow you to consume a good amount of each while still practicing weight management, and because of their low-fat and high-nutrient content, green fruits and veggies can help lower the risk of heart disease. Their nutrients can also help to facilitate your body's repair mechanism and protect you against free radicals, which contribute to the aging process and the formation of some cancers. Research shows that eating one serving of green vegetables a day can also help lower the risk of diabetes.

Selections from the green fruits and vegetables color list include:

- Avocados
- Apples
- Grapes
- Honeydew
- Kiwi
- Limes
- Pears
- Artichokes
- Arugula
- Asparagus
- Broccoli
- Brussels sprouts
- Green beans
- Celery
- Cucumbers
- Endive
- Kale
- Leeks
- Lettuce
- Green onions
- Okra
- Green peas
- Green peppers
- Snow peas
- Spinach

- Sugar snap peas
- Watercress
- Zucchini

A light snack throughout the day can not only help to boost, support, and maintain milk supply, but can help to balance energy and caloric intake. Opt for nutritious lactogenic super food combinations such as:

- Greek yogurt and granola paired with blueberries, strawberries, raspberries, or cherries
- Carrot sticks and celery served with lightened-up ranch dip
- A serving of fruit (grapes, honeydew, kiwi, or green apple) and nuts (raw almonds or walnuts)
- Sliced avocado on toasted whole grain bread
- Cucumbers marinated in vinegar
- A simple smoothie
- 1 cup of black tea and 2 no-bake energy bites
- 1 granola bar and a glass of milk
- Simple veggie salsa and baked tortilla chips
- A small spinach and kale side salad tossed with cucumbers, onions, peppers, celery, carrots, and tomatoes, and served with your favorite dressing.
- Fruit salad made with green fruits from the selection listed above.

You can also sprinkle snacks and salads with sesame, poppy, fenugreek, pumpkin, or sunflower seeds for a flavorful milk booster, or include brewer's yeast, flax seed, and/or oat straw in baked goods, quinoa, oatmeal, teas, and smoothies.

Tea Time

There are many popular lactation teas available on the market, including Mother's Milk Tea, which has been produced and sold since 1974. Whether these teas actually "work" to promote lactation depends on who you ask. Often, these teas are more beneficial to women who have already begun to produce breast milk than for those who hope to jump start lactation--and you have to drink a lot of it to optimize its success. I can't offer an honest opinion on this because, aside from home-blended brews, I've never tried a lactogenic tea. I do know that an effective and less experience alternative is black Oolong tea. That's it! You can use it as a base for herbal lactogenics, but it works very well on its own (and it's recommended for daily use during 30 Days of Inducing.)

Why Establishing a 30-Day Supplement Routine is So Important

Our bodies have a way of adapting to things, have you ever noticed that? We can acclimate to almost anything, until it finally becomes our "normal"--and this includes the use of herbal supplements. Over time, when our bodies have become too comfortable with them, galactagogues can lose their effectiveness, and might need to be substituted with a different lactogenic.

But not at first.

We read so much about the wonders of fenugreek (as well as blessed thistle and goat's rue) that they almost seem like magic in a bottle. Dreams of full, flowing breasts fill our minds, and after we've taken them with little (or no) results--or at least the results we were hoping for--we begin to feel disappointed and discouraged. The truth is, these herbs can take some time to "work"; they have to move into our bloodstream, release into our system, and our bodies have to adapt to them--and this happens differently for every woman.
Basically, while we're doing our thing, we have to let the supplements do their thing!! And we may not realize that they are...it's just taking some time.

It can take up to 6 weeks to determine if herbal supplements are effective, and to work, they have to be taken properly, in the right combination and does. For example, fenugreek has to be taken regularly and faithfully; if it isn't, it can actually cause a decrease in milk supply. It's also one of those herbs that you can't just quit taking cold turkey. It requires something of a weaning process. In some ways, herbal supplements require almost as much of a commitment as other forms of inducing.

During 30 Days of Inducing, I recommend that you select the herbal supplement (or combination of supplements) that you feel comfortable using, and take them exclusively for the entire 30 days. This should give you time to determine if they're working. Take them faithfully without altering them in any way, and commit to them, even if they don't seem to be effective. You might be surprised by what you find at the end of the month.
If you notice that you are having any adverse reactions to the supplements, discontinue use, and be sure that any herbal supplements you take are compatible with any prescription medications you are currently taking.

Here are some galactagogue combination suggestions that might be helpful. They all work a little differently, and like a lot of things, herbs are something of a trial and error process. More information on each herb (and many others) as well as dosage, preparation methods, and home-blended teas can be found in *A Fountain of Gardens.*

.Three Sisters Cocktail

☐ 1 fenugreek capsule
☐ 1 blessed thistle capsule
☐ 1 goat's rue capsule

Take this capsule cocktail 3 times a day before meals.

You can safely take 1-2 alfalfa capsules with this if you want to.

Simple Three Sisters Lactation Tea

Empty the contents of 1 fenugreek capsule, 1 blessed thistle capsule, 1 goat's rue capsule, and 1 alfalfa leaf capsule into a cup and add 6-8 ounces of boiling water. Allow the mixture to steep for several minutes before drinking. You can drink 3-5 cups of this tea per day.

Because blessed thistle is defined as a "bitter", it needs to taste bitter to be completely effective, so sweeten this tea as lightly as possible.

Golden Lady Cocktail 1

☐☐ 1 fenugreek capsule

☐☐1 alfalfa capsule
☐☐1 blessed thistle capsule

Take this capsule cocktail 3 times a day before meals.

Golden Lady Cocktail 2

☐☐1 dandelion leaf capsule
☐☐1 marshmallow root capsule
☐☐1 red clover capsule

Take this capsule cocktail 3 times a day before meals.

Golden Lady Cocktail 3

☐1 fenugreek capsule
☐1 blessed thistle capsule
☐1 red clover capsule

Take this capsule cocktail 3 times a day before meals.

The Mix and Match List:

You can create your own Golden Lady Cocktail by combining any of the following galactagogues, but take NO MORE THAN 9 CAPSULES PER DAY.
An example of mixing and matching would be to take 2 fenugreek and 1 alfalfa capsule 3 times per day or 2 blessed thistle and 1 red clover capsule 3 times per day.   Whatever you choose to combine, try the blend for an entire month and gauge your body's reaction and response to it.

1. Fenugreek (up to 2 capsules when combined with another supplements, up to 3 capsules when taken alone, 3 x per day)
2. Alfalfa (up to 2 capsules when combined with another supplement, up to 3 capsules when taken alone, 3 x per day)
3. Blessed Thistle (up to 2 capsules when combined with another supplement, up to 3 capsules when taken alone, 3 x per day)
4. Dandelion Leaf (up to 2 capsules when combined with another supplement, up to 3 capsules when taken alone, 3 x per day)
5. Marshmallow Root (up to 2 capsules when combined with another supplement, up to 3 capsules when taken alone, 3 x per day)
6. Red Clover (up to 2 capsules when combined with another supplement, up to 3 capsules when taken alone, 3 x per day)

ONLY combine goat's rue with fenugreek and blessed thistle.

30 Days of Inducing includes 7 plans, and because they rotate by week, it is better to begin the program on the first day of any calendar month that contains at least 30 days. Each day of inducing coincides with a specific plan, which is clearly notated to make your personal journey go as smoothly as possible.

It can be very helpful to make notes of your daily inducing routine (including times, as well as any supplements, breast boosters, or other adjustments you've made to the protocol) and track your progress. This simple reference will allow you to easily determine what is working--and what might need a bit of tweaking. 30 Days of Inducing includes a Personal Notes section for your convenience!

And, now, for the question that I'm asked most often by women as they prepare to begin one of the most uncertain, exciting, and rewarding journeys of their lives...

How much milk will I make?

This depends. Lactation is as unique as the individual who hopes to induce it. From drops to spoonfuls, every woman's experience will be different. And it will be wonderful. Your body will determine how much milk is "right" for you. Stay focused and positive, knowing that you are making progress in your own way.

So, now that we've covered the basics, let's get started with 30 Days of Inducing! I wish you great success in your journey into lactation.

With warmth and affection,

Jennifer Elisabeth Maiden
The Loving Milk Maid

Plan 1

Throughout the course of 30 Days, you will follow this guideline on days number 1, 8, 15, 22, and 29.

In the morning with breakfast:

- Take your first dose of supplements
- Take 1 pre-natal vitamin
- Drink 1 cup of black tea

With lunch:

- Take your second dose of supplements
- Drink 1 cup of black tea

In mid or late afternoon:

- Enjoy a light lactation-boosting snack
- Drink 1 cup of black tea

In the evening, with dinner:

- Take your third dose of supplements
- Drink 1 cup of black tea

For the Adult Nursing Couple:

- Nurse a minimum of once today.
- Perform today's massage technique a minimum of one time.
- Perform today's pumping technique a minimum of one time.

Substitution:

- If you do not plan to pump, replace today's pumping session with a second manual massage.

For the Occasional Nurser:

- Nurse a minimum of once today.
- Perform today's massage technique a minimum of one time.
- Perform today's pumping technique a minimum of one time.

Substitution:

- If this a nursing "off day", replace today's suckling session with an additional manual massage or pumping session. If you do not plan to pump, simply massage instead.

For the Self-Inducing Woman:

- Perform today's pumping technique a minimum of 2 times.
- Perform today's massage technique a minimum of one time.

Inducing To-Dos:

- Remember your scheduled set times.
- Several minutes before each inducing routine, drink 4 ounces of water. Immediately following the session, drink an additional 4 ounces.
- During nursing, be sure to use the proper latch and correct suckling techniques. Breast compressions can be added to this session.

Today's Massage Technique:

The Breastfeeding Massage

1. Begin on the right side, using your right hand, and place it, palm down, just below your collarbone.
2. Using firm pressure, in small circular motions, massage your way downward, along the entire breast, toward the nipple. Remember to massage the areola, too!
3. Once you have reached your nipple, begin to massage upward, using the same firm pressure and small circular motions.
4. When you have reached the top of your right breast, massage horizontally, toward the left armpit.
5. Once you've reached your underarm, cover the top of your right hand with the palm of your left hand, and begin to massage downward once more, just as you did in Step 2.
6. When you have reached the nipple of your left breast, repeat Steps 1-5, massaging the right breast for a total of 15 minutes.
7. Rest briefly if necessary, and then repeat Steps 1-5, massaging the left breast for a total of 15 minutes.

Today's Pumping Technique:

Power Pumping

With a double pump kit:

1. Choose a 1-hour block of time.
2. Pump for 20 minutes. Rest for 10 minutes.
3. Pump for 10 minutes. Rest for 10 minutes.
4. Pump for 10 minutes.
5. Finish.

With a single pump kit:

1. Choose a 1-hour block of time.

2. Pump one breast for 10 minutes. Rest for 5 minutes.
3. Pump the same breast for 5 minutes. Rest for 5 minutes.
4. Again, pump on the same side for 5 minutes.
5. Finish
6. Repeat Steps 2-5 on the opposite breast.

Throughout the Day:

- Drink enough water throughout the day to assure proper hydration, which helps with the milk-making process. To determine how much water your body requires, divide your weight in half, and drink the number in fluid ounces.
- Do your best to eat enough calories to encourage lactation and maintain supply.

Optional Addition:

- Add one topical breast booster to your inducing routine.

Optional Inducing Method:

- You may consider using a TENS Unit to provide additional stimulation throughout the day.

Before bed:

- Enjoy 1 cup of black tea

Always remember to:

- Stay relaxed
- Remain focused and positive
- Care for your breasts
- Get plenty of restNOTES:

Plan 2

Throughout the course of 30 Days, you will follow this guideline on days number 2, 9, 16, 23, and 30.

In the morning with breakfast:

- ☐ Take your first dose of supplements
- ☐ Take 1 pre-natal vitamin
- ☐ Drink 1 cup of black tea

With lunch:

- ☐ Take your second dose of supplements
- ☐ Drink 1 cup of black tea

In mid or late afternoon:

- ☐ Enjoy a light lactation-boosting snack
- ☐ Drink 1 cup of black tea

In the evening, with dinner:

- ☐ Take your third dose of supplements
- ☐ Drink 1 cup of black tea

For the Adult Nursing Couple:

- ☐ Nurse a minimum of once today.
- ☐ Perform today's massage technique a minimum of one time.
- ☐ Perform today's pumping technique a minimum of one time.

Substitution:

- If you do not plan to pump, replace today's pumping session with a second manual massage or traditional nursing session.

For the Occasional Nurser:

- ☐ Nurse a minimum of once today.
- ☐ Perform today's massage technique a minimum of one time.
- ☐ Perform today's pumping technique a minimum of one time.

Substitution:

- If this a nursing "off day", replace today's suckling session with an additional manual massage or pumping session.

For the Self-Inducing Woman:

- ☐☐Perform today's pumping technique a minimum of 2 times.
- ☐☐Perform today's massage technique a minimum of one time

Inducing To-Dos:

- ☐Remember your scheduled set times.
- ☐Several minutes before each inducing routine, drink 4 ounces of water. Immediately following the session, drink an additional 4 ounces.
- ☐During nursing, be sure to use the proper latch and correct suckling techniques. Breast compressions can be added to this session.

Optional Inducing Method:

- You may consider using a TENS Unit to provide additional stimulation throughout the day.
- You may include 1 round of nipple stimulation prior to any inducing method.

Today's Massage Technique:

The Areolae Massage

1. Begin on the right side.
2. Cover your areola with the flat of your hand, fingers pointing downward, and center your nipple against your palm.
3. Press inward firmly, pulling your breast against the wall of your chest, and begin to massage the areola in smooth, small, counter-clockwise circles. Be sure to move your entire breast and not just your hand when performing this effective inducing technique.
4. Massage in this manner for 5 minutes.
5. Massage the left breast, following Steps 2-4, and then return to the right breast.
6. Continue to perform areolae massage until you have stimulated each breast for a total of 15 minutes.

Note: If you would like to use areolae massage more often throughout the day you can do so by performing this technique every 3-4 hours.

Today's Pumping Technique:

Power Pumping

With a double pump kit:

1. Choose a 1-hour block of time.
2. Pump for 20 minutes. Rest for 10 minutes.

3.   Pump for 10 minutes. Rest for 10 minutes.
4.   Pump for 10 minutes.
5.   Finish.

With a single pump kit:

1.   Choose a 1-hour block of time.
2.   Pump one breast for 10 minutes. Rest for 5 minutes.
3.   Pump the same breast for 5 minutes. Rest for 5 minutes.
4.   Again, pump on the same side for 5 minutes.
5.   Finish
6.   Repeat Steps 2-5 on the opposite breast.

Throughout the Day:

● Drink enough water throughout the day to assure proper hydration, which helps with the milk-making process. To determine how much water your body requires, divide your weight in half, and drink the number in fluid ounces.
● Do your best to eat enough calories to encourage lactation and maintain supply.

Before bed:

● Enjoy 1 cup of black tea

Always remember to:

● Stay relaxed
● Remain focused and positive
● Care for your breasts
● Get plenty of rest

Plan 3

Throughout the course of 30 Days, you will follow this guideline on days number 3, 10, 17, and 24.

In the morning with breakfast:

- Take your first dose of supplements
- Take 1 pre-natal vitamin
- Drink 1 cup of black tea

With lunch:

- Take your second dose of supplements
- Drink 1 cup of black tea

In mid or late afternoon:

- Enjoy a light lactation-boosting snack
- Drink 1 cup of black tea

In the evening, with dinner:

- Take your third dose of supplements
- Drink 1 cup of black tea

For the Adult Nursing Couple:

- Nurse a minimum of once today.
- Perform today's massage technique a minimum of one time.
- Perform today's pumping technique a minimum of one time.

Substitution:

- If you do not plan to pump, replace today's pumping session with a second manual massage or nursing session.

For the Occasional Nurser:

- Nurse a minimum of once today.
- Perform today's massage technique a minimum of one time.
- Perform today's pumping technique a minimum of one time.

Substitution:

- If this a nursing "off day", replace today's suckling session with either an additional manual massage or pumping session.

For the Self-Inducing Woman:

- ☐ Perform today's pumping technique a minimum of 2 times.
- ☐ Perform today's massage technique a minimum of one time

Inducing To-Dos:

- ☐ Remember your scheduled set times.
- ☐ Several minutes before each inducing routine, drink 4 ounces of water. Immediately following the session, drink an additional 4 ounces.
- ☐ During nursing, be sure to use the proper latch and correct suckling techniques. Breast compressions can be added to this session.

Optional Inducing Methods:

- ☐ You may include 1 round of nipple stimulation prior to any or all inducing method(s).
- ☐ A TENS Unit can be used to provide additional stimulation throughout the day.

Today's Massage Technique:

Deep Tissue Massage

1. .Begin on the right side.
2. Using your right hand, firmly grasp your breast in a cradled C hold, as if you are performing compressions.
3. Press inward firmly, pulling your breast against the wall of your chest, and begin to massage in a downward stroking motion, as if you are expressing milk. Your fingers will help to support and compress the underside of your breast as your thumb presses gently inward in sliding circular motions.
4. Continue to stroke downward to the areola. As you stroke and compress, use the fingertips of your left hand to press firmly against the entire areola, massaging in small clockwise circles. Perform 2 rotations.
5. Continue to perform deep tissue massage in this way until you have stimulated each breast for a total of 15 minutes.

Note: If you would like to use this technique more often throughout the day you can do so by performing deep tissue massage every 3-4 hours.

Today's Pumping Technique:

Traditional Pumping

Pump each breast for a total of 20 minutes. It is often helpful to begin each pumping session with a five-minute rapid cycle (typically 70 on an electric pump, and in massage mode if your pump offers this feature) with a medium to high suction. (Choose a vacuum level that is approximately half of maximum suction to trigger let-down and simulate suckling.) Then, switch to expression mode, using your preferred level of suction for the remaining 15 minutes.

Optional Pumping Tips:

1. When you have finished the 15 minutes of pumping, set your pump on let-down/massage mode once more for an additional 5 minutes to ensure complete and proper milk removal.
2. Perform pump compressions
3. You may use Power Pumping in place of traditional pumping.

Throughout the Day:

- Drink enough water throughout the day to assure proper hydration, which helps with the milk-making process. To determine how much water your body requires, divide your weight in half, and drink the number in fluid ounces.
- Do your best to eat enough calories to encourage lactation and maintain supply.

Before bed:

- Enjoy 1 cup of black tea

Always remember to:

- Stay relaxed
- Remain focused and positive
- Care for your breasts
- Get plenty of rest

Plan 4

Throughout the course of 30 Days, you will follow this guideline on days number 4, 11, 18, and 25.

In the morning with breakfast:

- ☐ Take your first dose of supplements
- ☐ Take 1 pre-natal vitamin
- ☐ Drink 1 cup of black tea

With lunch:

- ☐ Take your second dose of supplements
- ☐ Drink 1 cup of black tea

In mid or late afternoon:

- ☐ Enjoy a light lactation-boosting snack
- ☐ Drink 1 cup of black tea

In the evening, with dinner:

- ☐ Take your third dose of supplements
- ☐ Drink 1 cup of black tea

For the Adult Nursing Couple:

- ☐ Nurse a minimum of once today.
- ☐ Perform today's massage technique a minimum of one time.
- ☐ Perform today's pumping technique a minimum of one time.

Substitution:

- If you do not plan to pump, replace today's pumping session with a second manual massage or nursing session.

For the Occasional Nurser:

- ☐ Nurse a minimum of once today.
- ☐ Perform today's massage technique a minimum of one time.
- ☐ Perform today's pumping technique a minimum of one time.

Substitution:

- If this a nursing "off day", replace today's suckling session with an additional manual massage or pumping session. If you do not plan to pump, use manual massage instead.

For the Self-Inducing Woman:

- ☐ Perform today's pumping technique a minimum of 2 times.
- ☐ Perform today's massage technique a minimum of one time

Inducing To-Dos:

- ☐ Remember your scheduled set times.
- ☐ Several minutes before each inducing routine, drink 4 ounces of water. Immediately following the session, drink an additional 4 ounces.
- ☐ During nursing, be sure to use the proper latch and correct suckling techniques. Breast compressions can be added to this session.

Optional Inducing Methods:

- ☐ You may include 1 round of nipple stimulation prior to any or all inducing method(s).
- ☐ A TENS Unit can be used to provide additional stimulation throughout the day.

Optional Addition:

- ☐ Add one topical breast booster to your inducing routine.

Today's Massage Technique:

Marmet

1. Position the thumb (above the nipple) and first two fingers (below the nipple) about 1" to 1–1/2" from the nipple, though not necessarily at the outer edges of the areola. Use this measurement as a guide, since breasts and areolae vary in size from one woman to another. Be sure the hand forms the letter "C" and the finger pads are at 6 and 12 o'clock in line with the nipple. (Do not cup your breast.)
2. Push straight into the chest wall. (Keep your fingers together, and if you have large breasts, first lift and then push into the chest wall.)
3. Roll your thumb and fingers forward at the same time. This rolling motion compresses and empties the milk reservoirs without injuring delicate breast tissue.
4. Repeat this rhythmic pattern to completely drain the breasts: Position, push, roll. Position, push, roll.
5. Rotate the thumb and fingers to milk other reservoirs, using both hands on each breast.
6. Avoid squeezing the breasts, sliding your hands over the breasts, or forcefully tugging on the nipples.
7. When you have performed Marmet on the first breast, move to the opposite side and repeat steps 1-5.

You can perform multiple sets of the Marmet Technique on each breast, spending 10-15 minutes per side.

Note: If you would like to use this technique more often throughout the day you can do so by performing Marmet every 3-4 hours.

Today's Pumping Technique:

Traditional Pumping

Pump each breast for a total of 20 minutes. It is often helpful to begin each pumping session with a five-minute rapid cycle (typically 70 on an electric pump, and in massage mode if your pump offers this feature) with a medium to high suction. (Choose a vacuum level that is approximately half of maximum suction to trigger let-down and simulate suckling.) Then, switch to expression mode, using your preferred level of suction for the remaining 15 minutes.

Optional Pumping Tips:

1. When you have finished the 15 minutes of pumping, set your pump on let-down/massage mode once more for an additional 5 minutes to ensure complete and proper milk removal.
2. Perform pump compressions.
3. You may replace power pumping for traditional pumping.

Throughout the Day:

*   Drink enough water throughout the day to assure proper hydration, which helps with the milk-making process. To determine how much water your body requires, divide your weight in half, and drink the number in fluid ounces.
*   Do your best to eat enough calories to encourage lactation and maintain supply.

Before bed:

*   Enjoy 1 cup of black tea.

Always remember to:

*   Stay relaxed
*   Remain focused and positive
*   Care for your breasts
*   Get plenty of rest

Plan 5

Throughout the course of 30 Days, you will follow this guideline on days number 5, 12, 19, and 26.

In the morning with breakfast:

- ☐ Take your first dose of supplements
- ☐ Take 1 pre-natal vitamin
- ☐ Drink 1 cup of black tea

With lunch:

- ☐ Take your second dose of supplements
- ☐ Drink 1 cup of black tea

In mid or late afternoon:

- ☐ Enjoy a light lactation-boosting snack
- ☐ Drink 1 cup of black tea

In the evening, with dinner:

- ☐ Take your third dose of supplements
- ☐ Drink 1 cup of black tea

For the Adult Nursing Couple:

- ☐ Nurse a minimum of once today.
- ☐ Perform today's massage technique a minimum of one time.
- ☐ Perform today's pumping technique a minimum of one time.

Substitution:

- If you do not plan to pump, replace today's pumping session with a second manual massage or traditional nursing session.

For the Occasional Nurser:

- ☐ Nurse a minimum of once today.
- ☐ Perform today's massage technique a minimum of one time.
- ☐ Perform today's pumping technique a minimum of one time.

Substitution:

- If this a nursing "off day", replace today's suckling session with an additional manual massage or pumping session. If you do not plan to pump, manual stimulation can be substituted.

For the Self-Inducing Woman:

- ☐ Perform today's pumping technique a minimum of 2 times.
- ☐ Perform today's massage technique a minimum of one time

Inducing To-Dos:

- ☐ Remember your scheduled set times.
- ☐ Several minutes before each inducing routine, drink 4 ounces of water. Immediately following the session, drink an additional 4 ounces.
- ☐ During nursing, be sure to use the proper latch and correct suckling techniques. Breast compressions can be added to this session.

Optional Inducing Methods:

- ☐ You may include 1 round of nipple stimulation prior to any or all inducing method(s).
- ☐ A TENS Unit can be used to provide additional stimulation throughout the day.

Today's Massage Technique:

Chi Breast Massage

1. Place your right hand over your right breast and your left hand over your left breast.
2. Spread your fingers out slightly and try to cover as much of your breast as possible.
3. Move your breasts inward, in a circular motion. Begin by moving the breasts toward one another, as if to create cleavage. Then, move them down and out, away from each other, and then up and toward each other again. This is one full rotation.
4. Perform 180-360 inward rotations.

Note: Because it is so effective, it should only be necessary to perform Chi a maximum of two times today. Allow at least 1 hour in between sessions to maximize effectiveness.

Today's Pumping Technique:

Traditional Pumping

Pump each breast for a total of 20 minutes. It is often helpful to begin each pumping session with a five-minute rapid cycle (typically 70 on an electric pump, and in massage mode if your pump offers this feature) with a medium to high suction. (Choose a vacuum level that is approximately half of maximum suction to trigger let-down and simulate suckling.) Then, switch to expression mode, using your preferred level of suction for the remaining 15 minutes.

Optional Pumping Tips:

1. When you have finished the 15 minutes of pumping, set your pump on let-down/massage mode once more for an additional 5 minutes to ensure complete and proper milk removal.
2. Perform pump compressions
3. You may use Power Pumping in place of traditional pumping.

Throughout the Day:

- Drink enough water throughout the day to assure proper hydration, which helps with the milk-making process. To determine how much water your body requires, divide your weight in half, and drink the number in fluid ounces.
- Do your best to eat enough calories to encourage lactation and maintain supply.

Before bed:

- Enjoy 1 cup of black tea

Always remember to:

- Stay relaxed
- Remain focused and positive
- Care for your breasts
- Get plenty of rest

Plan 6

Throughout the course of 30 Days, you will follow this guideline on days number 6, 13, 20, and 27.

In the morning with breakfast:

- ☐ Take your first dose of supplements
- ☐ Take 1 pre-natal vitamin
- ☐ Drink 1 cup of black tea

With lunch:

- ☐ Take your second dose of supplements
- ☐ Drink 1 cup of black tea

In mid or late afternoon:

- ☐ Enjoy a light lactation-boosting snack
- ☐ Drink 1 cup of black tea

In the evening, with dinner:

- ☐ Take your third dose of supplements
- ☐ Drink 1 cup of black tea

For the Adult Nursing Couple:

- ☐ Nurse a minimum of once today.
- ☐ Perform today's massage technique a minimum of one time.
- ☐ Perform today's pumping technique a minimum of one time.

Substitution:

- If you do not plan to pump, replace today's pumping session with a second manual massage or traditional nursing session.

For the Occasional Nurser:

- ☐ Nurse a minimum of once today.
- ☐ Perform today's massage technique a minimum of one time.
- ☐ Perform today's pumping technique a minimum of one time.

Substitution:

- If this a nursing "off day", replace today's suckling session with an additional manual massage or pumping session. If you do not plan to pump, manual stimulation can be substituted.

For the Self-Inducing Woman:

- ☐ Perform today's pumping technique a minimum of 2 times.
- ☐ Perform today's massage technique a minimum of one time

Inducing To-Dos:

- ☐ Remember your scheduled set times.
- ☐ Several minutes before each inducing routine, drink 4 ounces of water. Immediately following the session, drink an additional 4 ounces.
- ☐ During nursing, be sure to use the proper latch and correct suckling techniques. Breast compressions can be added to this session.

Optional Inducing Methods:

- ☐ You may include 1 round of nipple stimulation prior to any or all inducing method(s).
- ☐ A TENS Unit can be used to provide additional stimulation throughout the day.

Today's Massage Technique:

TCM Acupressure

1. STEP ONE: Point #1

To perform this point, you will use your thumbs to apply gentle pressure to the center of your chest. To find this point, it might be helpful to envision two straight lines: one will stretch from one nipple to the other, the second will run vertically down the center of your body. You will apply pressure where the strings intersect. Press this point five times.

2. STEP TWO: Point #2

To perform this point, you will use your thumbs to apply gentle pressure to the area beneath the breasts. To find this point, simply follow the nipple downward, to the area where the breast connects to the chest wall. Press this point five times on each side.

Note: Because TCM Acupressure is a highly effective manual technique, it should only be necessary to perform it a maximum of two times today. Allow at least 1 hour in between sessions to maximize effectiveness.

Today's Pumping Technique:

Traditional Pumping

Pump each breast for a total of 20 minutes. It is often helpful to begin each pumping session with a five-minute rapid cycle (typically 70 on an electric pump, and in massage mode if your pump offers this feature) with a medium to high suction. (Choose a vacuum level that is approximately half of maximum suction to trigger let-down and simulate suckling.) Then, switch to expression mode, using your preferred level of suction for the remaining 15 minutes.

Optional Pumping Tips:

1. When you have finished the 15 minutes of pumping, set your pump on let-down/massage mode once more for an additional 5 minutes to ensure complete and proper milk removal.
2. Perform pump compressions.
3. You may use Power Pumping in place of traditional pumping.

Throughout the Day:

- Drink enough water throughout the day to assure proper hydration, which helps with the milk-making process. To determine how much water your body requires, divide your weight in half, and drink the number in fluid ounces.
- Do your best to eat enough calories to encourage lactation and maintain supply.

Before bed:

- Enjoy 1 cup of black tea

Always remember to:

- Stay relaxed
- Remain focused and positive
- Care for your breasts
- Get plenty of rest

Plan 7

Throughout the course of 30 Days, you will follow this guideline on days number 7, 14, 21, and 28.

In the morning with breakfast:

- ☐ Take your first dose of supplements
- ☐ Take 1 pre-natal vitamin
- ☐ Drink 1 cup of black tea

With lunch:

- ☐ Take your second dose of supplements
- ☐ Drink 1 cup of black tea

In mid or late afternoon:

- ☐ Enjoy a light lactation-boosting snack
- ☐ Drink 1 cup of black tea

In the evening, with dinner:

- ☐ Take your third dose of supplements
- ☐ Drink 1 cup of black tea

For the Adult Nursing Couple:

- ☐ Nurse a minimum of once today.
- ☐ Perform today's massage technique a minimum of one time.
- ☐ Perform today's pumping technique a minimum of one time.

Substitution:

- If you do not plan to pump, replace today's pumping session with a second manual massage or traditional nursing session.

For the Occasional Nurser:

- ☐ Nurse a minimum of once today.
- ☐ Perform today's massage technique a minimum of one time.

- ☐Perform today's pumping technique a minimum of one time.

Substitution:

- If this a nursing "off day", replace today's suckling session with an additional manual massage or pumping session. If you do not plan to pump, manual stimulation can be substituted.

For the Self-Inducing Woman:

- ☐Perform today's pumping technique a minimum of 2 times.
- ☐Perform today's massage technique a minimum of one time

Inducing To-Dos:

- ☐Remember your scheduled set times.
- ☐Several minutes before each inducing routine, drink 4 ounces of water. Immediately following the session, drink an additional 4 ounces.
- ☐During nursing, be sure to use the proper latch and correct suckling techniques. Breast compressions can be added to this session.

Optional Inducing Methods:

- ☐You may include 1 round of nipple stimulation prior to any or all inducing method(s).
- ☐A TENS Unit can be used to provide additional stimulation throughout the day.

Today's Massage Technique:

The Doe Massage

1. Place your right hand on the inner side of your right breast and your left hand on the inner side of your left breast.
2. Move your hands down and then up, around the outer side of each breast until they reach the tops, and then move your hands back to the center of your chest. This is one full rotation. Imagine drawing a circle around your breasts; this is the motion you will be performing.
3. Perform 36 full rotations.

Note: This highly effective massage can be performed up to two times today, once in the morning and then again at night. Do 36 full rotations during each session. When performing The Doe, your hands will brush gently against the breasts; they will be the only thing that moves. Try not to shift your breasts in any way.

Today's Pumping Technique:

Traditional Pumping

Pump each breast for a total of 20 minutes. It is often helpful to begin each pumping session with a five-minute rapid cycle (typically 70 on an electric pump, and in massage mode if your pump offers this feature) with a medium to high suction. (Choose a vacuum level that is approximately half of maximum suction to trigger let-down and simulate suckling.) Then, switch to expression mode, using your preferred level of suction for the remaining 15 minutes.

Optional Pumping Tips:

1. When you have finished the 15 minutes of pumping, set your pump on let-down/massage mode once more for an additional 5 minutes to ensure complete and proper milk removal.
2. Perform pump compressions.
3. You may use Power Pumping in place of traditional pumping.

Throughout the Day:

- Drink enough water throughout the day to assure proper hydration, which helps with the milk-making process. To determine how much water your body requires, divide your weight in half, and drink the number in fluid ounces.
- Do your best to eat enough calories to encourage lactation and maintain supply.

Before bed:

- Enjoy 1 cup of black tea

Always remember to:

- Stay relaxed
- Remain focused and positive
- Care for your breasts
- Get plenty of rest

Conclusion
Day 31 and Beyond

Congratulations! You have completed 30 Days of Inducing. I hope you enjoyed this month-long program, and have found success in using it. Long-term lactation, which involves supply maintenance and building, requires much more than an initial 30 day commitment; to keep that liquid gold flowing, you'll need to continue to practice the daily inducing routine you've now established, and that is where the 30 Days of Inducing program transitions into the 30 Days of Maintenance program, and here are some tips on how to easily use it.

1. .Continue to induce one month at a time. Day 31 will begin the first day of Month 2.
2. Use the exact set inducing times you established during the initial 30 days.
3. This is the perfect time to determine if the herbal supplements you selected during 30 Days of Inducing are working for you. If they seem to be effective, continue to use them. If you're ready for a change, make the switch now, and use your new herbal combinations for a 30-day period of time.
4. You can follow 30 Days of Inducing as it is written as a means of supply building and/or maintenance, or select specific routines that you find most effective. Just remember to induce on schedule, and continue to follow the proper suckling, massage, and pumping patterns that you've grown familiar with.
5. To build and maintain supply, you'll need to induce or express at least once a day.
6. If you are building (and have not yet produced enough milk to physically express it by hand or with a breast pump), you'll need to induce a minimum of 27 out of 30 days. You can allow yourself up to 3 "free days" per month, but will need to induce for 9 consecutive days before taking a day off. Unless it's absolutely necessary, don't schedule your free days back to back. This can harm your supply.
7. Do what you're doing, and then do it again...and again...and repeat.
8. Stay positive, focused, and motivated--and if you need support or encouragement, join the 30 Days of Inducing group on the Bountiful Fruits forum!

I wish you great success and all the best in everything that you dream of achieving!

But we aren't done yet! Keep reading for 30 Days of Lactation Recipes, a selection of favorite DIY boobie boosters, my top breast pump picks, and tips on how to properly care for your beautiful new nursing breasts!

30 Days of Lactation Recipes

LMM's Breast Boosting Oatmeal
Servings: 1

Ingredients:

- 1 cup cooked oats
- 1/4 cup almond milk
- 1 tablespoon brewer's yeast
- 1 tablespoon flax seed
- 1 tablespoon flaked coconut
- 1 tablespoon raisins
- 1 tablespoon raw almonds, chopped
- Honey, to taste

Directions:

1. Sprinkle brewer's yeast and flax seed meal over warm oatmeal.
2. Gently stir in almond milk.
3. Fold in almonds and raisins. Top with coconut and drizzle with honey to taste.
4. Serve and enjoy!

Loving Milk Maid's All-Time Favorite Granola
Servings: 3 1/2 cups

Ingredients:

- 3 cups old-fashioned oats
- 1 tablespoon kosher salt
- 1 tablespoon cinnamon
- 1/3 cup honey
- 1/4 cup sunflower oil
- 2 teaspoons pure vanilla extract

Directions:

1. Preheat your oven to 300 degrees F.
2. .In a large bowl, combine oats, kosher salt, and ground cinnamon. Set aside
3. .In a separate bowl, blend together raw honey, sunflower oil, and vanilla.

4. Pour the honey and oil mixture into the dry ingredients and combine well until the oats are completely coated.
5. Spread the granola into a 9 x 13 ungreased baking dish and bake on the center rack of your preheated oven for 15 minutes.
6. After 15 minutes, stir granola and continue baking for an additional 5-15 minutes, or until it is lightly golden brown. Do not overbake; it will continue to bake and set in the pan once it is removed from the oven.
7. Place pan on a wire baking rack and allow granola to cool completely before transferring it to an airtight container.

Peanut Butter and Jelly Smoothie
Serves: 1

Ingredients:

- ☐ 1 cup milk
- ☐ 1 1/2 cups fresh or frozen blueberries, thawed
- ☐ 1 tablespoon flax seed meal'
- ☐ 2 teaspoons oat straw powder
- ☐ 2 tablespoons peanut butter

Directions:

1. Add all ingredients to your blender. Simply blend until smooth.
2. Serve and enjoy!

Go Green Salad
Servings: 1

Ingredients:

- ☐ 1/2 cup lettuce, roughly torn
- ☐ 1/2 cup spinach, roughly torn
- ☐ 1/2 cup broccoli florets
- ☐ 1/2 cup artichoke hearts
- ☐ 1/2 avocado, chopped
- ☐ 1/2 stalk celery, diced
- ☐ 1 green onion, chopped

Directions:

1. Toss all ingredients together in a salad bowl. Sprinkle with salt and pepper to taste.
2. Serve with your favorite dressing and enjoy!

Simple Vinaigrette
Servings: 1

Ingredients:

- ☐ 3 tablespoons extra-virgin olive oil
- ☐ 1 tablespoon apple cider vinegar

- Pinch of salt
- Pinch of black pepper

Directions:

1. Add all ingredients to a small bowl.
2. Whisk until well blended.
3. Serve with your favorite salad and enjoy!

Cherry Walnut Oatmeal
Servings: 1

Ingredients:

- 1 cup cooked oatmeal
- 3 tablespoons vanilla Greek yogurt
- 1/2 cup fresh cherries, chopped
- 1 tablespoon walnuts, chopped
- 2 teaspoons honey

Directions:

1. Stir yogurt into warm oatmeal. Top with cherries. Drizzle with honey and sprinkle with chopped walnuts.
2. Serve and enjoy!

Caprese Salad for One
Servings: 1

Ingredients:

- 1 1/2 cups tomatoes (plum, cherry, and grape), chopped
- 1 ounce mozzarella cheee, cubed
- 1/2 teaspoon extra-virgin olive oil

Directions:

1. Place chopped tomatoes in a bowl. Drizzle with olive oil.
2. Add cubed cheese, and toss lightly to coat.
3. Allow the Caprese to marinate for a few minutes before sprinkling with salt and dried basil to taste.
4. Serve and enjoy!

Flourless Pumpkin Bread
Servings: 1 loaf

Ingredients:

- 2 cups old-fashioned oats
- 1/2 cup honey
- 15 ounces canned pumpkin

- ☐ 2 eggs
- ☐ 1 teaspoon baking soda
- ☐ 1 teaspoon pumpkin pie spice
- ☐ Dash of vanilla extract

Directions:

1. Preheat your oven to 350 degrees F. Prepare a loaf pan with nonstick cooking spray.
2. Add all ingredients to a blender and mix until well blended and smooth, pausing to scrape sides of blender when necessary.
3. Pour batter evenly into prepared loaf pan.
4. Bake for 30-45 minutes, or until a toothpick inserted in the center of the bread comes out clean. Begin checking your bread at the 30-minute mark to avoid over-baking.
5. Allow bread to cool completely in the pan before slicing and serving.

The Green Monkey Smoothie
Servings: 1

Ingredients:

- ☐ 1 cup almond milk
- ☐ 2 tablespoons almond butter
- ☐ 1 tablespoon coconut oil
- ☐ 1 tablespoon brewer's yeast
- ☐ 1 tablespoon flax seed meal
- ☐ 1 tablespoon oats, uncooked
- ☐ 2 teaspoons oat straw powder
- ☐ 2 cups spinach, finely chopped
- ☐ 1 banana, sliced
- ☐ 2 teaspoons honey

Directions:

1. Add all ingredients to a blender. Blend until smooth.
2. Serve and enjoy!

Light and Fit Ranch Dip
Servings: 4

Ingredients:

- ☐ 2 tablespoons dried parsley
- ☐ 1 1/2 teaspoons dried dill weed
- ☐ 2 teaspoons garlic powder
- ☐ 2 teaspoons onion powder
- ☐ 2 teaspoons onion flakes
- ☐ 1 teaspoon black pepper
- ☐ 1 teaspoon dried chives
- ☐ 1 teaspoon salt
- ☐ 8-ounce container plain nonfat Greek yogurt

Directions:

Blend the dry ingredients together in a small bowl.
Add 3 tablespoons of dry mix to the yogurt, stirring well to incorporate, and allow the dip to rest in the fridge for 30 minutes before serving.
To prepare 1 serving of dip, add 1 tablespoon of dry seasoning mix to 1/4 cup yogurt.
Leftover dry mix can be stored in an airtight container for up to 3 months.

Coconut Chai Spice Oatmeal

Servings: 1

Ingredients:

- 1 cup cooked oatmeal'
- 1/4 cup almond milk
- 2 tablespoons flaked coconut
- 2 teaspoons brown sugar
- 1/4 teaspoon cinnamon
- 1/8 teaspoon ginger
- Pinch of nutmeg
- Pinch of cloves
- Pinch of ground cardamom
- Pinch of black pepper

Directions:

1. Prepare 1 cup of oatmeal, and allow to set for 2-3 minutes.
2. Stir in almond milk, and then add other ingredients, mixing until well-blended.
3. Serve and enjoy!

Savory Curry Quinoa
Servings: 1

Ingredients:

- 1 cup cooked quinoa
- 1/2 cup coconut milk
- 1 tablespoon green onions
- 1 tablespoon coconut oil
- 1/4 teaspoon ginger
- 1/4 teaspoon garlic powder
- Pinch of tumeric
- Pinch of coriander
- Pinch of cumin
- Pinch of cardamom
- Pinch of cayenne pepper

Directions:

1. Prepare 1 cup of quinoa and transfer to a bowl.

2. Gently stir in the milk, and then add the remaining ingredients, mixing until well incorporated.
3. Serve and enjoy!

Peaches and Cream Smoothie
Servings: 1

Ingredients:

- ☐ 3/4 cup almond milk
- ☐ 1/2 cup vanilla Greek yogurt
- ☐ 1 ripe peach, fresh or frozen, thawed
- ☐ 1 tablespoon brewer's yeast
- ☐ 1 tablespoon flax seed meal
- ☐ 2 teaspoons oat straw powder
- ☐ 1/8 teaspoon pure vanilla extract
- ☐ 2 teaspoons honey

Directions:

1. Add all ingredients to you blender. Blend until smooth.
2. Serve and enjoy!

Traditional Lactation Cookies
Servings: 5 dozen

Ingredients:

- ☐ 1 cup butter
- ☐ 1 cup granulated sugar
- ☐ 1 cup brown sugar, firmly packed
- ☐ 2 eggs
- ☐ 1 teaspoon vanilla extract
- ☐ 3 cups all-purpose flour
- ☐ 2 tablespoons flax seed meal
- ☐ 4 tablespoons brewer's yeast
- ☐ 1 teaspoon baking soda
- ☐ 1 teaspoon salt
- ☐ 3 cups quick-cooking oats
- ☐ 1 cup chocolate chips

Directions:

1. Preheat your oven to 350 degrees Farenheit.
2. In a large mixing bowl, using an electric mixer, cream together the butter and sugars. Add the eggs one at a time, mixing well after each addition. Stir in the vanilla.
3. Mix in the dry ingredients, stirring until well-incorporated.
4. Fold in the chocolate chips.
5. Scoop cookie dough into tablespoon-sized balls and drop onto ungreased cookie sheets. Bake for 10-12 minutes. Allow cookies to rest on baking sheets for 1-2 minutes before transferring to wire cooling racks.

Carrot Apple Slaw
Servings: 4-6

Ingredients:

- 1 large red apple, julienned
- 1 Granny Smith apple, julienned
- 3 cups carrots, julienned
- 1/4 cup raisins
- 1/4 cup golden raisins
- 1/3 cup vanilla Greek yogurt
- 1/3 cup plain Greek yogurt
- 1 tablespoon lemon juice
- 2 tablespoons honey
- 2 teaspoons apple cider vinegar
- Salt, to taste

Directions:

1. In a mixing bowl, toss julienned apples in lemon juice. Add carrots and stir to combine. Set aside.
2. In a separate bowl, whisk together the yogurt, honey, vinegar, and salt. Pour the dressing over the slaw mixture and stir until well coated.
3. Fold in the raisins.
4. Refrigerate for at least 30 minutes before serving.

Gingerbread Smoothie

Servings: 1

Ingredients:

- 1 3/4 cups almond milk
- 2 ripe bananas, sliced
- 1 teaspoon ginger
- 1 teaspoon cinnamon
- 1/2 teaspoon pure vanilla extract
- 2 tablespoons molasses
- 1 tablespoon flax seed meal
- Flaked coconut, optional

Directions:

1. Add all ingredients to a blender. Mix until smooth. Top with flaked coconut for additional flavor.
2. Serve and enjoy!

Simple Tomato Salad
Servings: 1

Ingredients:

- ☐ 1 cup cherry tomatoes, halved'
- ☐ 1/8 teaspoon garlic powder
- ☐ 1 teaspoon dried basil
- ☐ 2 teaspoons balsamic vinegar
- ☐ 1 tablespoon olive oil
- ☐ Salt to taste

Directions:

1. Toss tomatoes in herbs, oil, and vinegar until evenly coated.
2. Sprinkle with salt and pepper to taste.
3. Serve immediately and enjoy!

Oatmeal Pancakes
Servings: 12 pancakes

Ingredients:

- ☐ 1/2 cup all-purpose flour
- ☐ 1/2 cup quick-cooking oats
- ☐ 1 teaspoon granulated sugar
- ☐ 1 teaspoon baking powder
- ☐ 1/2 teaspoon baking soda
- ☐ 1/2 teaspoon salt
- ☐ 3/4 cup buttermilk
- ☐ 1 teaspoon pure vanilla extract
- ☐ 2 tablespoons sunflower oil
- ☐ 1 egg

Directions:

1. Whisk all ingredients together in a large mixing bowl until well-blended.
2. Heat a lightly oiled skillet over medium-high heat. Pour 1/4 cup of pancake batter into a circle in the skillet. When the batter begins to set around the edges and bubbles appear on the surface, flip the pancake over. Cook for an additional 1-2 minutes, or until completely done.
3. Repeat with remaining batter.
4. Serve and enjoy!

Asparagus with Lemon Sauce
Servings: 4

Ingredients:

- ☐ 20 asparagus spears
- ☐ 1/4 cup plain Greek yogurt
- ☐ 1 teaspoon dried dill
- ☐ 2 tablespoons lemon juice
- ☐ Pinch of sugar
- ☐ Salt and black pepper to taste

Directions:

1. Steam the asparagus spears until crisp-tender and easily pierced with the tines of a fork.
2. While the asparagus is steaming, whisk together the yogurt, lemon juice, dill, sugar, salt, and pepper until well-blended.
3. Spoon lemon sauce over cooked asparagus spears.
4. Serve and enjoy!

Cranberry Sauce
Servings: 4

Ingredients:

- 4 cups cranberries
- 1/2 cup unsweetened applesauce
- 1 cup orange juice
- 1/3 cup agave syrup
- 1/2 teaspoon cinnamon
- 1/4 teaspoon cloves
- 1/4 teaspoon nutmeg

Directions:

1. Place cranberries, applesauce, orange juice, and agave in a medium saucepan.
2. Bring to a boil over medium heat. Reduce to simmer and add spices.
3. Let simmer for 10-12 minutes, or until most of the cranberries burst.
4. Remove from heat and allow to cool completely before serving.

Red Velvet Smoothie Bowl
Servings: 1

Ingredients:

- 1 banana, frozen and sliced
- 1/2 cup beets, frozen and chopped
- 1/4 cup vanilla Greek yogurt
- 2 tablespoons cacao powder
- 1/4 cup coconut milk

Optional Toppings:

- Sliced strawberries
- Cacao nibs
- Whipped cream

Directions:

1. In a blender, mix together the first 5 ingredients and transfer to a bowl.
2. Top with sliced berries, whipped cream, and chopped cacao nibs.
3. Serve and enjoy!

Apple Pie Breakfast Porridge
Servings: 1

Ingredients:

- 1 cup cooked quinoa
- 1 small apple, peeled, cored, and finely chopped
- 1 teaspoon cinnamon
- 3/4 cup almond milk
- 1/4 teaspoon nutmeg
- 2 tablespoons maple syrup

Directions:

1. Add maple syrup to warm cooked quinoa and allow to set for 3-5 minutes.
2. n a medium bowl, combine apples, cinnamon, and nutmeg, and microwave on high for 2 minutes, or until apples have become slightly tender.
3. Top the quinoa with spiced apples and almond milk. Garnish with chopped walnuts if desired.
4. Serve and enjoy!

Carrot Cake Overnight Oats
Servings: 1

Ingredients:

- 1/2 cup oats
- 3/4 cup almond milk
- 1/4 cup carrots, grated
- 1 tablespoon maple syrup
- 1/4 teaspoon vanilla
- 1/2 teaspoon cinnamon
- 1/8 teaspoon ginger
- 2 tablespoons raisins
- 1/4 cup walnuts, chopped

Directions:

1. In a bowl, combine all ingredients, stirring until well-blended.
2. Cover and refrigerate overnight.
3. In the morning, give the oats a quick stir. Serve and enjoy!

Sparkling Cranberry Limeade Mocktail
Servings: 6

Ingredients:

- 5 ounces frozen limeade concentrate
- 64 ounces cranberry juice
- 2 liter sparkling lemon-lime water

Optional Garnish

- ☐Fresh cranberries
- ☐Lime slices

Directions:

1. Add frozen limeade to a large pitcher.
2. Stir in cranberry juice.
3. Add sparkling water.
4. our mocktail into glasses garnished with fresh cranberries and lime slices.
5. Serve and enjoy!

Gingerbread Pancakes
Servings: 12 pancakes

Ingredients:

- ☐2 eggs
- ☐1/4 cup molasses
- ☐2 cups buttermilk
- ☐1/2 tablespoon baking powder
- ☐2 cups all-purpose flour
- ☐1/2 teaspoon baking soda
- ☐1/2 teaspoon salt
- ☐1 teaspoon ginger
- ☐1 teaspoon cinnamon
- ☐1/2 teaspoon nutmeg
- ☐1/4 teaspoon allspice

Directions:

1. In a large bowl, whisk together eggs, molasses, and buttermilk. Set aside.
2. In a separate bowl, mix all dry ingredients until well combined.
3. Slowly add the dry mixture to the wet ingredients, whisking just until all ingredients are combined.
4. Lightly oil a skillet and heat over medium heat. Pour 1/4 cup pancake batter into a circle and cook for 2-3 minutes or until air bubbles form on the surface. Flip and cook for an additional 3-5 minutes.
5. Repeat with remaining batter.
6. Serve with your favorite toppings and enjoy!

Spiced Blueberry Mango Smoothie
Servings: 1

Ingredients:

- ☐1/2 cup blueberries, frozen
- ☐1/2 cup mango, frozen
- ☐1/2 teaspoon ginger
- ☐1/2 tablespoon tumeric

- ☐ 1 teaspoon orange juice
- ☐ 1/2 tablespoon apple cider vinegar
- ☐ 1/2 tablespoon coconut oil
- ☐ 3/4 cup almond milk
- ☐ Pinch of black pepper, optional

Directions:

1. Place all ingredients in a blender, and blend until smooth and creamy.
2. Serve and enjoy!

Mixed Berry Banana Smoothie Bowl
Servings: 1

Ingredients:

- ☐ 1 cup almond milk
- ☐ 1 cup mixed berries (blueberries and raspberries)
- ☐ 1 banana, sliced
- ☐ 1/3 cup fresh spinach
- ☐ 1/2 teaspoon pure vanilla extract
- ☐ 2 tablespoons flax seed meal

Optional Garnish:

- ☐ 1/2 cup strawberries, sliced
- ☐ 1/2 banana, sliced
- ☐ 1/4 cup granola

Directions:

1. Add all ingredients to a blender and mix until smooth. Transfer to a bowl.
2. Garnish with strawberries, sliced bananas, and granola.
3. Serve and enjoy!

Sunshine Rice
Servings: 4

Ingredients:

- ☐ 1 cup brown rice
- ☐ 1 1/2 tablespoons olive oil
- ☐ 1 1/4 cups celery, finely chopped
- ☐ 1 1/4 cups white onion, finely chopped
- ☐ 1 cup water
- ☐ 1/2 cup orange juice
- ☐ 2 tablespoons lemon juice

Directions:

1. In a large pan over medium-high heat, warm the olive oil. Add celery and onions and cook until tender, about 10 minutes.
2. Add water and citrus juices to pan and bring to a boil.
3. Stir in rice. Reduce heat and cover pan with a lid. Simmer until all liquid is absorbed, approximately 20 minutes.
4. Remove pan from stove and allow rice to set for several minutes. Fluff with a fork. Serve and enjoy!

Three Bean Side Salad
Servings: 4-6

Ingredients:

- 2 cups green beans, fresh or frozen, cut into bite-sized pieces
- 2 cups lima beans
- 1 cup edamame
- 4 tablespoons vinegar
- 1/2 tablespoon granulated sugar
- Salt and black pepper to taste

Directions:

1. Bring a pot of water to boil over medium-high heat. Add lima beans and edamame, reduce heat, and simmer for 4-6 minutes, or until beans are tender.
2. Add green beans and cook for an additional 1-2 minutes.
3. Drain beans and rinse in cool water until they've reached room temperature. Set aside.
4. In a medium bowl, whisk together vinegar and sugar. Add beans, tossing lightly to coat. Season with salt and pepper.
5. Refrigerate for 30-60 minutes before serving.

The Ultimate Lactation Smoothie
Servings: 1

Ingredients:

- 1 1/2 cups raw spinach
- 1/2 cup cooked oatmeal
- 2 tablespoons brewer's yeast
- 2 tablespoons flax seed meal
- Cinnamon to taste
- 1 banana, sliced
- 1 green apple, finely chopped
- 1 cup black tea
- Several dashes of almond milk (if needed to thin the smoothie)

Directions:

1. Add all ingredients into a blender in the order listed above. If necessary to thin the smoothie, add a small amount of almond milk (or coconut water), and blend until thick and creamy.

2.   Serve and enjoy!

Loving Milk Maid's
Favorite DIY Boobie Boosters

Milk Mask Base

1/4 cup of powdered milk is all you need to make a fantastic mask base, which can be used to prepare a variety of custom-blended boobie boosters! Consider adding a few drops of essential oils, aloe vera, or your favorite carrier oil and just enough warm water to make a thick, but easy to spread paste. Once applied to the breasts, allow your milk mask to dry completely before rinsing with warm water.

Banana Mask

You will need:

- 1/4 cup yogurt
- 2 tablespoons honey
- 1 medium banana

Optional Ingredients:

- Essential oils
- Vitamin E oil

Directions:

Mash the banana, and stir in the yogurt and honey until smooth. Apply to the breasts and allow to set for 10-20 minutes before rinsing with warm water.

Avo-Coco Mask

You will need:

- 1/4 ripe avocado
- 1 tablespoon cocoa powder
- 1 tablespoon honey

Directions:

In a small bowl, mash the avocado, and then stir in the cocoa and honey until a thick paste is formed. Apply to the breasts and allow to set for 15 minutes before rinsing with warm water.

As a simple alternative, you can substitute the ripe avocado with 1 tablespoon of avocado oil.

Sour Cream Mask

You will need:

- 1/2 cup sour cream
- 1 egg yolk
- 2 teaspoons pure aloe vera juice or gel

Optional Ingredients:

- Essential oils
- 1 teaspoon Vitamin E oil

Directions:

Whisk all ingredients together in a small mixing bowl. Apply evenly to the breasts, and allow the mask to set for 30 minutes before rinsing with warm water.

As an alternative, you can substitute the sour cream with 1/4 cup powdered milk, and include 1 1/2 tablespoons of either apple cider vinegar or lemon juice to the recipe.

Loving Milk Maid's
Best Breast Pump List

Over the course of the past 28 months, ever since I began my journey into the Land of
Re-Lactation, I've learned a lot about breast pumps--not just about the pumps themselves,
but also about their efficiency, effectiveness, and the best way to use them as a method of
inducing lactation. If they aren't currently producing maternal breast milk, adult nursing
women have much different needs than lactating and/or breastfeeding mothers. For
instance, when first beginning the inducing process, you won't need to focus so much on
how effective a pump is at drawing milk from the breasts into a collection bottle (that will
come later), but how well it can stimulate the breasts to encourage milk production and
flow. Of course, as time goes by and you begin to actively lactate, you'll want a pump that
helps to maintain your supply by providing proper milk removal, so, basically, as an adult
nursing woman, you'll be looking for an "all in one" kind of pump to fulfill all of your
nursing needs without costing a small fortune.

There will always be debate over whether or not pumping "works" as an inducing method. I
was unsure of this, too, when I first began the process, but I now feel comfortable in being
able to say yes, I believe it does work, and as a matter of fact, I feel that it is much more
effective than previously thought. And, no matter what others may say, if you're
incorporating a great suckling session (or two) and at least one manual form of stimulation
into your daily inducing routine, you do not have to pump every two hours around the clock
to achieve lactation success. (And what a relief, because, let's be honest, who really has the
time for that?) Pumping schedules are another common topic for conflicting opinion, with
the belief that a pump must be utilized throughout the day--*and* night to maximize its
effectiveness. However, no matter what others may say, if you're incorporating a great
suckling session (or two) and at least one manual form of stimulation into your daily
inducing routine, you do not have to pump every two hours around the clock to achieve
lactation success. (And what a relief, because, let's be honest, who really has the time for
that?) Research has shown that the frequency of pumping does not determine lactation
success; it is better to allow our breasts to rest, rejuvenate, and replenish themselves to
encourage milk synthesis. Getting a good night's rest rather than waking up to pump
through the night actually *increases* our chance of making milk.

Over the past year, I've been doing a lot of research into the breast pump industry, and found that there are a lot (and by a lot, I mean hundreds) of pumps on the market, and each one has specific functions and features, and its own unique list of pros and cons, as well as mixed reviews on stimulation, expression, suction, and backflow. Breast pumps are really no different than any other product: they can't really be designed specifically for every woman's individual needs; they're just one of those things that you have to try for yourself to be able to determine how well it suits your body and lifestyle. This is kind of unfortunate because a good-quality breast pump is an investment, one that can cost anywhere from $100 to $500 (or more), and purchasing and replacing in the pursuit to find the perfect pump just isn't a realistic option for all of us.

When compiling my Best Breast Pump List, I gathered info provided by industry experts, spoke to various nursing women, visited lots of websites, made a few phone calls, and pored over thousands of reviews, and hope all of this will help you find the perfect pump! But before we explore my top pump picks, here are some things to know prior to making a final decision:

1. There are four type of breast pumps to consider:

- Hospital grade pumps are highest quality and generally termed "the most efficient" variety of pump because they are designed for multiple uses, making them a great choice for the inducing woman who is not yet lactating, or those who hope to increase their milk flow. Because they're double kit pumps, they allow you to pump both breasts at once, and accurately mimic suckling patterns, which can help greatly in the inducing process. Hospital grade pumps do cost a bit more than other styles, but many are reasonably priced.
- Electric pumps provide a high cyclic rate, which not only mimics proper suckling patterns, but also ensures faster stimulation and expression times. These double kits are especially good for women who are self-inducing and plan to pump more frequently, those who are only able to nurse occasionally, and women who have currently established lactation and are able to draw milk from their breasts. Electric pumps are known to be portable, efficient, and fairly economical.
- Battery operated pumps are portable and lightweight, but have low cyclic rates. They will effectively stimulate one breast at a time, and can be used to induce, but are more effective if used along with other traditional inducing methods such as suckling and/or manual massage. These are often used by nursing women who do not currently need to express milk, and prefer not to use a manual pump. Battery operated pumps are very cost-efficient, too.
- Manual pumps can be used to induce alongside other forms of traditional inducing. Along with being extremely inexpensive, they are lightweight, easy to store, take up very little space, and very portable. Manual pumps are a great choice for women who are just starting out, to determine if pumping is going to be an option for them, those who hope to build and/or maintain their milk supply at a slower pace, and as a way to ease nursing breast discomfort. Cyclic rate will depend on your ability to pump.

2 Phases and Modes:

Consider investing in a breast pump that offers various phases and modes; these are sometimes known as 2-Phase Expression Mode(s). This will help you to imitate terrific and effective suckling patterns that stimulate (or massage) the breasts to trigger let-down prior to milk ejection (expression).

3. Pump Kits:

Most breast pump systems include a pump kit, which often contains at least 1 (and sometimes 2 in various sizes) set of flanges/breast shields, applicable pump parts (such as tubing and valves), and collection bottles. It's nice to have the opportunity to test out different flange sizes to determine what works perfectly for you. Generally, pump kits include the industry standard sized shields (24 mm), and often 1 larger (28 mm) pair, too. Don't be surprised if you need a different sized flange for each breast; this is not an uncommon occurrence.

4. Backflow Protection:

Sometimes, moisture builds up in pump tubing, which can cause bacteria and viruses to spread. Pumps with backflow protection prevent this and provide a hygienic pumping experience. If you do notice moisture in your tubing, you can leave your pump on for a few minutes after you've finished inducing to dry it.

5. Comfort:

Pumping should never be painful, and since breast pumps are often a big part of the inducing process, selecting one that is comfortable to use can be an important part of the selection process. Many companies now label their systems as being "comfortable"--and this comfort actually depends on the flange design. If you feel uncomfortable, some brands offer breast shield inserts to make the pumping process more pleasant.

Pumping Tips:

1. Be sure your breast shields fit correctly. Your nipple should be centered in the flange tunnel, and move freely when your pump is turned on. It shouldn't rub against the flange walls, and you shouldn't feel pinching or compression. If your flange is too big, you may notice that your pump draws a lot of your breast into the tunnel, and this will make for ineffective stimulation.
2. Don't pump too hard; inducing is much more effective if you pump at your maximum level of comfort. If you notice any discoloration or feel any discomfort, you might be pumping too forcefully.
3. More isn't always better, so try to pump each breast for a maximum of 20 minutes. This allows them time to rest and replenish...and they may just be more willing to cooperate with you during their next pumping session! :)
4. Practice with your pump's phases and modes and suction to find what feels good--and seems to be working for you!

When compiling my top picks list, I was looking for "all in one" pumps that would work very well for both inducing and expression, and would be compatible with all breasts and budgets. To make my list, a breast pump had to fulfill my personal Key E Requirement. They needed to be:

1. Effective
2. Efficient
3. Economical

I selected pumps that would be perfect for every day use, fulfill both traditional and Power Pumping needs, and withstand the test of time, so you'll get more "bang for your buck". (Which I think is important because a great pump is a true investment.)

I also paid close attention to ratings, grades, and reviews. None of my top picks received less than a 4 star rating, and none are priced higher than $300, which can still be fairly expensive, but is a lot more affordable than one industry recommended and top-rated Rolls Royce of Breast Pumps, which comes with not only a lot of fantastic features, but also the incredibly steep price tag of $2,000.

Just like everything else, nothing is perfect, so in this list, I was sure to note the "cons" right along with the "pros" to give a fair and honest assessment of each of these pumps. They are listed from highest rated and graded to lowest, but any of them would make a wonderful choice for your personal pumping needs!
And, now, without further delay, I present, for your consideration, my Best Breast Pump List!

1. Medela Pump in Style Advanced Breast Pump with On the Go Tote

Style:

Double pump kit

Includes:

- Tote with AC adapter
- 2 sizes of breast shields (24 mm and 27 mm)
- Collection bottles (5-ounce)
- Cooler bag and ice packs

Features:

- 2 phase pumping expression technology
- Attached to the included carry-all bag
- Easy to find replacement parts and accessories
- Extra large flanges are available to accommodate women with large breasts and/or nipples
- Strong suction to help maintain supply or a lighter suction option to maximize inducing
- Provides great mobility, and can be easily moved to various pumping areas
- Easy to clean
- Compatible with all standard sized collection bottles
- Fully adjustable vacuum and speed settings
- Efficient

Things to Consider:

- Open system does not provide backflow protection
- Noisy
- Heavy and not ideal for travel
- Expensive
- Flanges may leak

- Less suction control
- Battery pack sold separately
- Battery connection issues
- Car charger is sold separately

Average Price Range:

- $229-$250

2 Spectra Baby USA S2 Double/Single Electric Breast Pump

Style:

Double pump kit

Includes:

- 2 sizes of breast shields (24 mm and 27 mm)

Features:

- Great for establishing lactation and proper milk removal
- Lightweight, compact enough for on the go pumping
- Quiet
- Backflow filters
- Timer
- Night light
- Gentle with fully customizable speed, suction, and vacuum
- Massage mode works well to prompt let-down
- Comfortable
- Perfect for every day use
- Wonderful for all breast types
- Can be used as a double or single pump

Things to Consider:

- No battery or AC adapter
- Does not include a carrying case

Notes:

The Spectra S2 is compatible with Medela breast shields. It is recommended that you purchase a travel adapter for use with this model.

Average Price Range:

- $120-$170

3.Ameda Purely Yours Double Electric Breast Pump

Style:

Double pump kit

Includes:

- 4 collection bottles
- 3 sizes of breast shields

Features:

- Comfortable and effective
- Airlock system to prevent backflow and the spread of bacteria and viruses
- Small and portable
- Discreet pumping bag
- Includes a battery and AC adapter
- Things to Consider:
- Less power and less suction than some other electric models
- Expensive

Average Price Range:

- $245-$300

4. Medela Freestyle Hands Free Double Electric Breast Pump

Style:

Hands free, double pump kit

Includes:

- Cooler bag
- Ice packs

Features:

- Small and portable
- Hands free capability
- Includes a power cord and battery pack
- One-touch let-down
- Suction levels ranging from 1-9
- Lightweight and provides true mobility
- Timer
- Memory button

Things to consider:

- Light suction
- Expensive
- Hands free pumping can be very difficult until you find a position that works well for you.

Average Price:

- $300

5. BelleMa Double Electric Breast Pump

Style:

Double pump kit

Includes:

- 2 collection bottles
- 1 bottle adapter

Features:

- Gentle and hygienic
- Closed system to prevent backflow, which can spread bacteria and viruses
- Very comfortable
- 2-phase pumping
- Can be used as a double or single pump
- Extra-long and convenient power cord
- Left and right individual controls to adjust suction on each breast
- Weighs just 14 ounces
- Easy to assemble
- Moderately quiet
- Economical
- Easy to clean and dries quickly

Things to consider:

- Battery must be purchased separately
- No carrying case
- No pause button

Notes:

The included bottle adapter allows you to use Avent and Medela collection bottles with this BelleMa system. This particular pump is comparable to the Medela Pump in Style, and rated much better than the BelleMa Melon model.

Average Price Range:

- $99-$139

6. Lansinoh Affinity Double Electric Breast Pump

Style:

Double pump kit

Includes:

- Collection bottles
- Breast shields
- Milk storage bags

Features:

- Customizable vacuum strength and cycle speed
- Closed system to prevent backflow, which spreads bacteria and viruses
- Standard and large sized flanges are available
- Affordable
- Very few parts, which makes for easy assembly and clean up
- Hygienic
- Offers stimulation and expression modes
- Moderately quiet

Things to Consider:

- Suction is gentle, but not particularly strong

Average Price Range:

- $104-$130

7. Evenflo Advanced Double Electric Breast Pump

Style:

Double pumping kit

Includes:

- 2 collection bottles
- 3 sets of different sized breast shields

Features:

- Very affordable
- Easy to clean
- Closed system to prevent tubing backflow

Things to Consider:

- Loud/noisy

Notes:

This is a great pump to consider if you're unsure of how often you'll be pumping; it's economical enough to be a starter pump, too!

Average Price Range:

- $90-$110

8. Medela Harmony Manual Breast Pump

Style:

Single manual

Includes:

- 1 24 mm breast shield

Features:

- Inexpensive
- Portable and lightweight
- Discreet and perfect for pumping on the go
- Quiet and easy to use
- Gentle
- Comfortable, soft shields
- Manual 2-phase expression technology
- Very few parts, which makes for easy assembly and easy clean up

Things to Consider:

- It can sometimes be difficult to achieve great suction with this pump
- Tiring

Notes:

This pump is compatible with other Medela shields, making it very convenient to find replacement parts. For a manual model, it is very effective, and sufficient for daily inducing. If you notice that your pump begins to squeak, you may want to consider cleaning it, or tightening any loose parts; these things often help solve the problem!

Average Price Range:

- $29-$43

9. Philips Avent Manual Comfort Pump

Style:

Single manual

Includes:

- 1 standard breast shield

Features:

- Lightweight
- Small and compact
- Easy to position and use
- Shield includes a massaging cushion for comfort and better stimulation
- No excess parts
- Great for travel
- Helps to prevent hand strain
- Good for women with flat nipples
- Angled neck allows gravity to work with you to aid in milk flow
- Affordable
- Easy on the back because you don't need to lean forward to pump

Things to Consider:

- Hard to assemble
- Requires specific wide neck Avent bottles to work
- Milk may drip from beneath the shield cushion
- Can squeak, making it a bit less discreet
- You may need to press the flange fairly hard against the breast to achieve good suction

Notes:

Despite its cons, this inexpensive and effective manual pump really works to get the job done and is sufficient for daily inducing.

Average Price Range:

- $24-$44

Honorable Mention:

Lansinoh Signature Pro Double Electric Breast Pump

Style:

Double pumping kit

Includes:

- 2 collection bottles
- 2 25 mm flanges

Features:

- Lightweight and compact
- Affordable
- Three pump styles
- Eight adjustable suction levels
- Digital display
- Hygienic
- Closed system to prevent the backflow that can cause bacteria

Notes:

This pump runs on the included AC adapter or 6 AA batteries (not included)

Average Price Range:

- $100-$150

Lansinoh Manual Breast Pump

Style:

Single manual pump

Includes:

- 2 breast shields: 1standard size, 1 larger sized

Features:

- Compact and lightweight
- Quiet and discreet
- Great for travel and on the go pumping
- 2 phase manual pumping
- Affordable
- Easy to assemble and easy to clean
- Comfortable

Notes:

I used this pump during my early days of inducing, and found that it was very efficient. It fit my breasts comfortably, and I was pleased with both the suction and the soft, flexible flanges. Even with the specially designed comfort-grip handle, my hand and arm felt fatigued every time I induced; however, at one point during Mr. S' week-long absence, I was pumping 3 times a day, so it might be comfier if used less frequently. At the time, I was a large and full DDD cup size, but was still able to use the standard 25 mm flanges, although I did have to lean slightly into the pump to maximize efficiency.

Average Price Range:

- $29-$40

Loving Milk Maid's Breast Pump Top Pick:

Without question, my favorite breast pump (and personal choice for inducing) is the Spectra Baby USA S2 Double/Single Electric Breast Pump. There really isn't much that this versatile, all-purpose pump can't do! I highly recommend it for all of your inducing needs.

Loving Milk Maid Reviews:
Spectra S2 Double/Single Electric Breast Pump

When I was in search of the "perfect pump" to assist me on my journey into re-lactation, I found myself faced with the same dilemma as many other nursing women: oh, the options! So many pumps, and all of them promised to be the "best". I knew that a breast pump I selected would need to fit some very specific criteria:

1. Economical, so I could induce without breaking the bank.
2. Efficient, so I could induce as quickly as my schedule allowed.
3. Effective in both the re-lactation and milk removal process.

And I wasn't sure that one hospital-grade pump would be able to fill such a tall order.

But after doing quite a bit of research, reading through dozens of positive reviews, and receiving three glowing recommendations from fellow nursing women, I found exactly what I was looking for in my Spectra S2, and I could not be happier!

Over the past 25 months, my Spectra (which is privately known as Glinda, an homage to my favorite quote from The Wizard of Oz...you know the one: You've always had the power, my dear, you just had to learn it for yourself...) and I have become very well acquainted! (As a matter of fact, Mr. S calls her my "breast friend"...haha) It's all good. She's everything you'd want in a BFF: dependable and reliable with the uncanny ability to make you feel good all over. My Spectra S2 has been an invaluable part of my daily inducing routine, and is the first pump I've ever really enjoyed using.

I know how strange it must seem to read about one woman's unabashed love for a motorized piece of medical equipment, but until you've spent hours of your life working diligently to produce breast milk, you really can't understand the importance or value of a high-quality pump.

My Thoughts on the Spectra Baby USA Brand:

"Our pumps don't suck, they suckle!"
--Spectra Baby USA

How adorable is that for a Twitter tagline?

Spectra Baby USA is one of the top leading breast pump companies run by Registered Nurses and Board Certified Lactation Consultants, and the number one source for innovative, stylish, affordable, and extremely efficient pumps and accessories. They offer five breast pump options, including the "Handy Manual" (want to try!), a beautiful Bling Collection (Hello! Yes, please!), an assortment of accessories (including a tote bag and cute little pink cooler bag kit), and offer breast shield sets and flanges in four convenient sizes: S (20 mm), M (24 mm), L (28 mm), and XL (32 mm), so you'll be sure to find your perfect fit!
The company's website is easy to navigate and user-friendly. I've shopped online with Spectra several times, and have always been completely satisfied with my experience and purchases.

The breast pump industry is a big world, and companies are vying for your business; each brand strategically markets their products to their target audience...and why wouldn't they? After all, they have something they want to sell, and they hope it's something you'll want to buy. We're all looking for the best. So, how do I think Spectra Baby USA measures up to all they claim to offer?

Very, very well.

Their S2 is innovative and very sophisticated. I've used other pumps in the past (as a breastfeeding mother rather than a nursing wife), and, to be honest, I always felt as if I were hooked up to some sort of milking machine. It was a noisy (and sometimes completely uncomfortable) experience. Until the Spectra S2 came into my life, I was a very indifferent pumper. Now, I can honestly say that I love to pump with a purpose.

Yes, their products are affordable. (The Bling Collection is a bit pricier, of course, but what can we expect from a custom made pump absolutely covered with genuine Swarovski crystals? *Adding to wish list*) Because of this pump's all-in-one features and functions, you get a lot of value for your money!

As for efficiency? 10/10.

And finally...here is a pump that doesn't suck. The suckling feature is fabulous, and as you're allowing the S2 to perform its milk making magic, it feels as if it's really getting the job done! Love it!

The bottom line?

I feel that the people at Spectra Baby USA not only recognize and understand the needs of the breastfeeding woman, but actually care about them, too.

12 Reasons Why I Love My Spectra S2:

1. Design

This pump is sleek, lightweight, and very compact. It provides a lot of mobility (which means you can pump anywhere, as long as there is an electrical outlet in close proximity), and the slim, curved handle makes it very easy to transport. While perhaps not considered a true on-the-go-travel-friendly pump, I've found that, when necessary, the Spectra S2 can be used as such, and is very easy to travel with! Glinda has now been on several family vacations, and she takes up very little room. Because I typically pump and dump when out and about, I did not invest in an insulated carry bag; my Spectra S2 fits comfortably in a sturdy average-sized tote bag, which provides a lot of discretion, and is easy to store. Aside from being practical, this pump is super-cute and pink! (Not that this really matters when it comes to efficiency and effectiveness, but I happen to like things that are aesthetically pleasing and pink, so it's a nice bonus, and if you're going to spend a lot of time with something, it might as well look nice, right?)

2. Digital Display with Timer

This is a very nice feature! The display is crisp, clear, and easy to read, showing the mode icon, cycle, and vacuum as you pump, and the built-in timer means no more clock-watching! The Spectra S2 keeps track of time for you!

3. Night Light

This is another one of those thoughtful little extras, courtesy of Spectra. The 2-level night light is bright without being overpowering, and easily allows you to pump under the cover of darkness.

4. 2 Phase Pumping

The Spectra S2 provides both massage (let-down) and expression mode, which means you'll be able to effectively induce and remove milk with one versatile pump! Massage mode is automatically set to a cycle of 70, which perfectly mimics the suckling performed during let-down that triggers milk ejection, and the vacuum can be adjusted from L1-L5. In this mode, you'll feel a gentle, but effective, fluttering against your breast. In expression mode, you can set your cycle speed to 38, 42, 46, 50, or 54, and choose from 12 levels of suction (L1-L12).

5. Fully Customizable

This is a fabulous feature because every woman is unique, and inducing works differently for all of us! The Spectra S2 allows you to customize the settings that work perfectly for you, in a combination of modes, cycles, and vacuum. This means you have complete control over your personal inducing and/or milk removal process!

6. Hygienic

This is a closed system with backflow protectors, which prevents milk and moisture from becoming trapped in the tubing (which can cause a build up of mold, bacteria, and other creepy-crawlies) and motor, which can ruin your unit.

7. Discreet

Unless you're using a manual model, no breast pump is completely soundproof--and some are super-noisy. The Spectra S2 is very quiet for an electric unit, and the motor runs very smoothly. It's provided me with hours of discreet pumping. (Very important to the adult nursing lifestyle!)

8. Easy to Assemble

When I first received my Spectra S2, I was concerned about putting it together, particularly the backflow protectors, but I soon realized that there wasn't anything to worry about! I was able to assemble everything (including the backflow membranes) in minutes. The included user manual is a big help: it's very straightforward and includes plenty of "how-to" diagrams.

9. Easy to Clean

Some of the parts are dishwasher safe, others need to be hand-washed in warm, soapy water. To clean the motor, all you have to do is wipe it down with a damp cloth.

10. Effective and Efficient

The Spectra S2 is a completely versatile pump, one I feel is effective for all nursing women, regardless of her state of lactation; it's perfect for aiding in establishing breast milk, and does a wonderful job of removing it, too, which helps to build and maintain supply. As a woman with large breasts, I've found that proper milk removal has been an issue in the past with other pumps, but I don't have this problem with my S2. The double pump feature makes this a very efficient way to induce and express when time is an issue, and using the Spectra S2 as a single pump kit allows you to be semi-hands free.

11. Durable

For a small and compact system that weighs just a little more than 3 pounds, this high-quality pump has substance! I've been using mine for a minimum of once a day for the past 2 years, and have now spent numerous hours power pumping with it, and my Spectra S2 is still going strong!

12. Comfortable

When using a breast pump as frequently as many inducing women do, comfort is a big issue. The S2 really is a "feel good" kind of pump. The breast shields are just flexible enough to mold comfortably to my breasts, creating a firm, but pain-free seal, that ensures optimum suction. When drawing milk from my breasts with other pumps, the pull was sometimes forceful and harsh, but with my Spectra S2, both the massage and expression modes provide deep, but extremely comfy, stimulation. (Yes, there are tingly feels involved, but they are really good feels! Trust me!)

What Others Have Said:

With every drop of sunshine there comes a little rain, and nothing is perfect, so to offer a fair and honest assessment of the Spectra S2, I'm going to address some of the "cons" commonly associated with this pump. (Note: these issues probably won't factor in quite as much for an adult nursing woman as they would for a breastfeeding mama.)

1. No battery

Spectra Baby USA offers the S1 model, which does include a built-in rechargeable battery. For a few extra dollars, you can experience the luxurious freedom of going sans power cord. (The S1 seems to provide the same fabulous features and functions as the S2; as well as having the built-in battery, it's cute and blue.)

2. Suction Issues

Some women feel that the S2's suction leaves a bit to be desired when the pump is used as a single kit. Personally, because of my daily schedule, I'm a double pumper, but I wanted to test this for myself. I didn't notice a difference in suction when I used the S2 as a single kit with my preferred settings. As long as the port cap is securely in place, I don't think this will be much of an issue. However, this may depend on personal suction preferences, and it may be helpful to adjust your settings when using the single pumping function.

3. No pump or carry-all bag

Spectra Baby USA offers a very stylish black tote for about $30, which can be used to store and transport your S2, but you won't be able to pump from inside of it, and it isn't roomy enough for a cooler kit. Because discretion is so important to me, the inability to be able to pump from a bag isn't a top concern, but if a pump bag is on your personal nursing checklist, this might be something to consider.

4. Finding the Sweet Spot

I feel that being fully customizable is a "pro" when it comes to the "perfect" pump, but some women think it's a little difficult to find their pumping sweet spot right away with the Spectra S2. This is probably because the pump offers an almost limitless number of adjustable mix-and-match variants to make the pumping experience ideal for every woman's individual needs. It can take some time to find the settings that work best for you, so just practice with them! Eventually (and probably sooner than you think), you'll find the sweet spot, and when you do...ah! Bliss!

If I Could Change One Thing About the Spectra S2, it Would Be...

The power cord. It's short. I found this out really early on. I was all set up in my cozy little pumping space and ready for action. Glinda began doing her thing, and I was really getting into the rhythm when I shifted slightly to the left, and, suddenly, everything just stopped. Was this a malfunction? I went into brief panic mode until I realized that I'd pulled the power cord from the outlet. I've had to make a few adjustments, and because I pump in the privacy of my bedroom, I have plenty of power source options. The short cord makes it more difficult when traveling because I have to determine the best areas to pump in more unfamiliar settings, but so far, everything's worked out pretty well. With that being said, a longer power cord is definitely on my Spectra S2 pump wish list.

My Final Thoughts:

The Spectra S2 is definitely an all-in-one pump, practical, affordable, and versatile enough to easily accommodate all nursing women's breasts and lifestyles!

Loving Milk Maid's Tips:
How to Use a Manual Breast Pump for Maximum Efficiency and Effectiveness

There is a wide selection of breast pumps available on the market, and nursing women have very discerning tastes when it comes to their particular pump of choice, often going to great lengths to find one that is perfectly suited to their particular needs. I found myself facing that same dilemma early into my non-maternal lactation journey. As a breastfeeding mother, I wasn't a huge breast pump fan, and I wasn't sure that I was going to pump within my ANR. I soon discovered, however, that pumping was actually going to be a necessity, so I began to look into pump options. I first chose a single manual pump before investing in a hospital-grade electric pump.

There is a lot of debate over the manual versus electric pump. Although electric pumps can be a lot more convenient for in-home use, they aren't always practical for active non-maternal nursing women on the go. Adult nursing is a private and discreet part of many couple's lives, and explaining why you're carrying an electric breast pump with you when there are obviously no little ones to sustain is simply not a viable option. Manual pumps take care of that problem; they are lightweight, easy to assemble, and can be discreetly stored away from prying eyes. And they are also much more economical than their electric counterparts.

Electric breast pumps can be expensive, ranging from about $179.00 upwards to $500.00 or more--and this price doesn't include a carrying case. The cost of investing in an electric breast pump just isn't in everyone's budget.
I do love my electric breast pump; it does a lot of the work for me, as I can efficiently pump both breasts at once, and set the controls to determine let-down stimulation, suckling stimulation, and my maximum comfort level, but, with that being said, I also found that my manual pump was a true lifesaver early on, and I'm really glad that I had it on hand. It did its job very well, and has actually worked quite well to collect milk now that I am fully lactated and actively producing.

I would suggest that women new to ANR first invest in a manual pump; you can sort of "test the waters" to determine if you'll enjoy pumping before making a very large purchase. Later, as you commit to the pumping process, begin to require more stimulation, or after you have begun to produce larger quantities of milk, you may want to consider investing in an electric model. To get started, a manual pump is really all that you'll need.

While it's true that breast pumps can provide very good stimulation to help with milk production, their main goal is actually to draw milk from the breast and collect it. That's why using a pump to encourage lactation needs to be done properly. Essentially, you want your breasts to believe that there is a need for all of that beautiful milk, and the best way to do that is to mimic the feeding pattern of an infant. You can do this easily with a manual breast pump.

Before I explain how to do this, I thought I would share a few tips with you.

1   Flange (or breast shield) size is very important. The rim of your shield needs to completely encircle your areola. If you have large breasts, you'll notice that there is quite a bit of uncovered breast on either side of the flange. (Mr. S and I tease, calling it "overspill" or "excess boobage") Don't worry--as long as your areola is covered, you'll be just fine.

- Your flange should not compress your breast by squeezing or pinching it; there should be no pain at all. You should only feel a deep pull against the breast.
- Your flange should not pull your areola or excess breast tissue into it, either. Once you have centered your nipple into the flange tunnel, it should move freely forward-- and it should be the only part of your breast inside that tunnel.

2.   Suction is another important part of using a manual pump properly. Some women pump harshly, and well over their maximum comfort level, believing that the forceful stimulation is necessary to efficient milk production. It isn't. Remember, vacuum is only used to collect breast milk; it really has nothing to do with making breast milk.

Something to avoid:

My breast shield always feels too tight, and I have trouble taking it off of my breast. I've been using Vaseline, and now, it slides right off.

A breast shield should fit snugly. If it feels too tight, as if its squeezing your breast, then it is probably either too small or you are pumping with too much force.

Petroleum jelly can damage the materials used to make breast shields, so I wouldn't suggest using it as a lubricant. It's important to remember to break your pump's suction before removing a flange from your breast. If you still feel that a lubricant is necessary, though, coconut oil is a better choice. It won't break down your flange, and it's very good for your breasts.

Most manual pumps are equipped with some sort of device (a lever or a button) that allows a woman to adjust the tension and resistance of her pump handle, which helps to either simulate the let-down reflex or suckling. My Lansinoh manual pump has a small white lever on the top of the handle; by sliding it back, I can simulate let-down. To trigger let-down, adjust your pump to its highest resistance level before you begin. When you do this, the handle will tighten.

On a manual pump, maximum comfort level is typically determined by how a woman depresses her pump handle. If you press the handle "all the way" into the pump's collection bottle, sometimes hearing the click of the contact, the suction will be much more forceful, and you will be pumping at maximum level. You don't need to do this unless you want to; your pump will work just as effectively if you only depress the handle halfway in. It isn't the force of the pumping, but the rhythm of the motions that is important.

When first put to the breast, an infant sucks very rapidly to encourage milk flow. These quick "pacifier sucks" offer no pause for a "swallow rest". Infants provide two sucks per second when attempting to trigger let-down.

To mimic this rhythm with your manual pump, you will need to depress the handle in quick, short repeated bursts. You can do this by counting "1-2, 1-2, 1-2" to easily time the rhythm. It will be a continuous motion, fast, but steady, and you'll need to repeat this for 3-5 minutes to ensure that let-down has occurred.

Manual pumps provide "comfort grip handles" to prevent hand and arm fatigue, but when you first begin manual pumping, no matter how "comfortable" that handle is, you'll feel the effects. It's strenuous to pump, but it gets a lot easier as your hands adapt to the motion. It's important to keep up that fast "1-2" let-down motion when pumping, but if you can't do it for five minutes without breaking, stop and rest for a minute or two, before picking up your rhythm once more. Just remember, the rest time doesn't count as active pumping time, so be sure to actively pump for 3-5 minutes.

When you have triggered let-down, you can adjust your pump's tension to simulate proper suckling. When I slide my pump's lever forward, the tension loosens and my handle becomes much easier to depress.
When a baby realizes that the time to actually eat has arrived, he slows his suckling to a content and leisurely rate, pausing to swallow in between sucks. Babies are so attuned to the breast that they will actually adjust their feeding rhythm to ensure maximum efficiency. They will often show a ratio of two sucks for every one swallow, or even three sucks per swallow.

To pattern this suck-swallow rhythm while using your manual pump, you will do this by depressing and then releasing your pump's handle. The two depresses represent "suck-suck", and the rest release represents "swallow". You can time the rhythm by repeating "1,2-rest...1-2-rest..." or "1-2-3-rest" as you pump. The depressions will be rapid; just as with let-down stimulation, you will still depress the handle twice (or even three times) per second, but the rest will last for approximately two seconds. You will need to continue this pattern for about 10-15 minutes, depending on the length of time you pumped to simulate let-down.

Be sure to pump each breast in the same way, for the same length of time to ensure proper stimulation.

Before you know it, you'll be a breast pumping pro!

Loving Milk Maid's Tip:
Proper Breast Care for the
Adult Nursing Woman

Breast care is a vital part of every woman's life, but it becomes even more important for the adult nursing woman, who can experience the same common maladies as a traditionally breastfeeding mother. Sore, dry, or cracked nipples, clogged milk ducts, engorgement, mastitis, and thrush can often be avoided, or prevented entirely, through employing a proper latch, using correct suckling techniques, and practicing good daily breast care.

Here are my tips to ensuring the health of your beautiful breasts!

Prior to every inducing or nursing session, bathe your breasts in warm water and a gentle, non-irritating soap. Rinse thoroughly and pat the entire breast dry with a soft towel. Be sure to remove all moisture.

Repeat this process after inducing and/or nursing. If you cannot bathe the breasts following a session, be sure to at least dry your nipples and areolae thoroughly, particularly if you'll be wearing a bra, as moisture encourages both irritation and the growth of bacteria.

Ensure that your nipples and areolae stay well hydrated by applying a lanolin based cream, lotion, or balm designed for the delicate tissue of the breasts.

Practice proper breast milk removal--and empty those breasts!

Avoid harsh soaps and lotions that may irritate and dry the breasts, areolae, and nipples.

Stay well-hydrated by drinking an adequate amount of water every day.

Perform frequent breast self-examinations.
Be sure to schedule your yearly mammogram!

By following these easy steps, nursing can be a beautiful, pleasant, and healthy experience!

PERSONAL NOTES

PERSONAL NOTES:

PERSONAL NOTES:

PERSONAL NOTES:

PERSONAL NOTES:

About The Author

Known to readers around the world as The Loving Milk Maid (or simply LMM), freelance writer and blogger Jennifer Elisabeth Maiden gained recognition with the launch of her original blog, Bountiful Fruits: A Loving ANR Journey, and now runs the successful websites Bountiful Fruits, which explores the fascinating world of the adult nursing relationship and provides visitors with information on lactation, breastfeeding, relationships, intimacy, sex, and marriage, and the natural lifestyle site, Loving Milk Maid's. Ms. Maiden is an ANR/ABR advocate and educator who believes in promoting positive body image, recognition of the beautiful female anatomy, and happily-ever-afters, and is the author of several books, including *The Art of Lactation* and *A Fountain of Gardens*. She and her husband, Mr. S, reside in Ohio where she is currently working on her

newest work